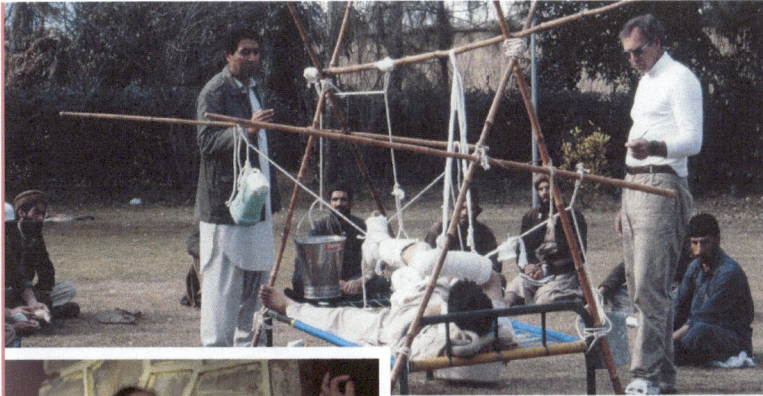

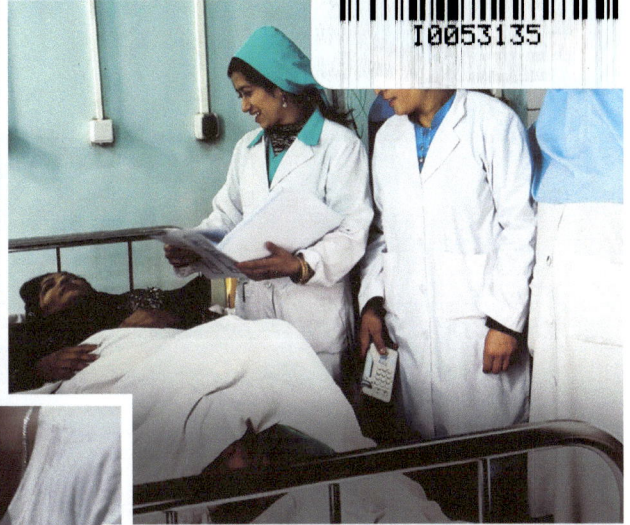

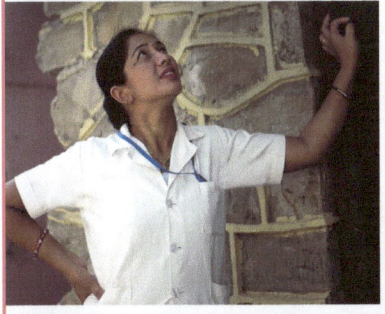

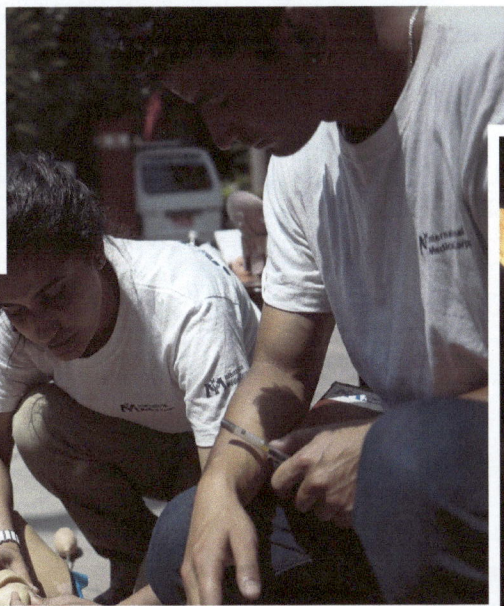

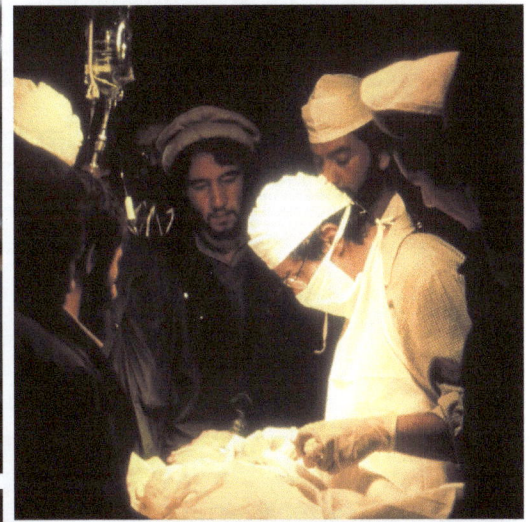

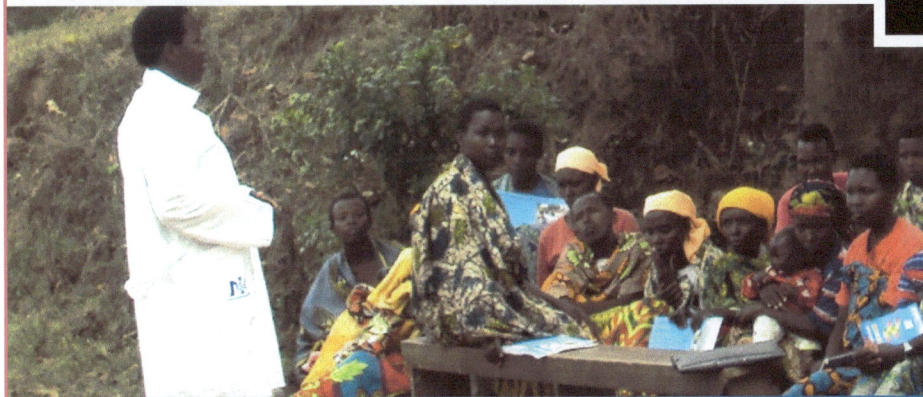

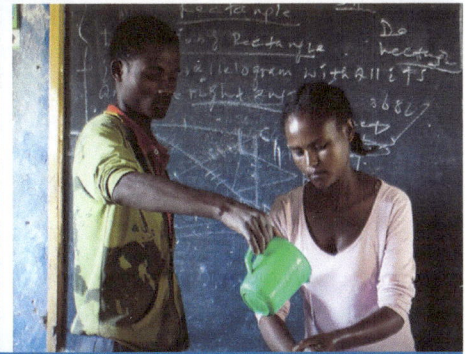

INTERNATIONAL MEDICAL CORPS

TRAINING MANUAL

EDITORS:

Robert R. Simon MD
Henry H. Hood MD

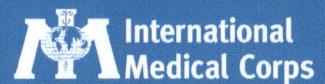

International Medical Corps

UNIT 1 Cardiology

International Medical Corps Training Manual

Unit One
Cardiology

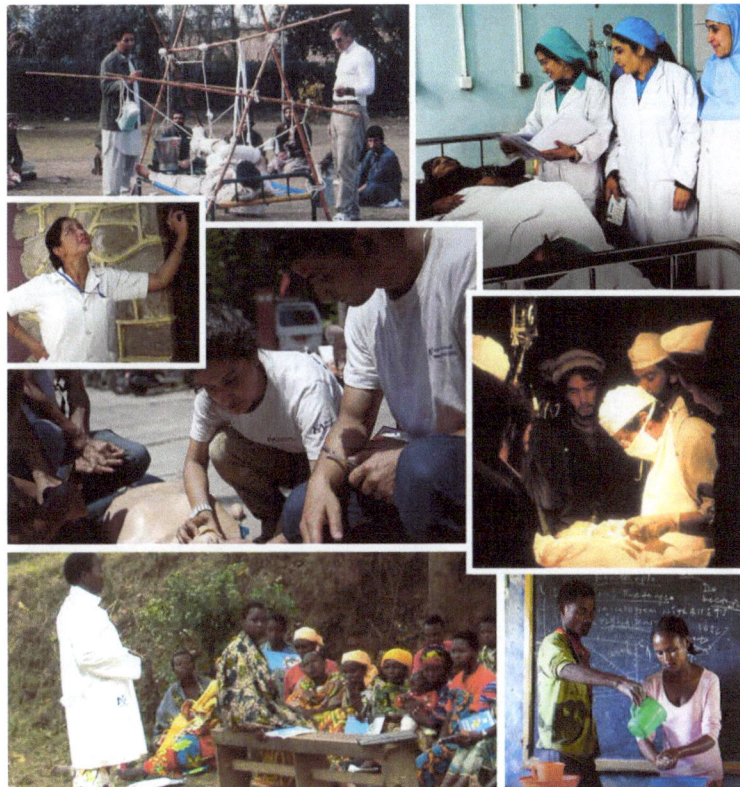

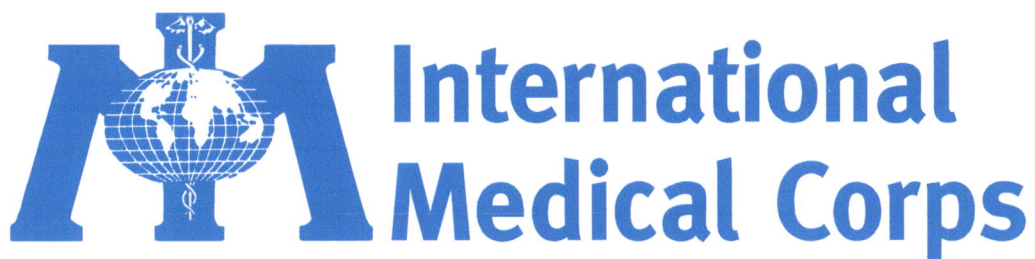

International Medical Corps

International Medical Corps Training Manual

Robert R. Simon MD
Henry H. Hood MD
Editors

Editorial Board:
Nancy Aossey

Visnja Cipcic

Bill Sundblad

International Medical Corps

www.internationalmedicalcorps.org

2017

Text © 2016 by International Medical Corps

Images © 2016 by International Medical Corps

Library of Congress Control Number: 2016933836

Manual ISBN 978-1-944812-00-3 (paper)

Manual ISBN 978-1-944812-18-8 (eBook)

UNIT 1 ISBN 978-1-944812-19-5 (paper)

UNIT 1 ISBN 978-1-944812-01-0 (eBook)

Printed in the United States of America.

First printing: April 2017

version 1.0.0

International Medical Corps
12400 Wilshire Blvd.
Suite 1500
Los Angeles, CA 90025
310-826-7800
www.internationalmedicalcorps.org

DEDICATION

This manual is dedicated to the members of the International Medical Corps family, numbering now in the thousands. Since our beginning, you have been courageous, diligent, inventive, and relentless. You have treated the sick and injured. Just as important you have taught, thereby multiplying International Medical Corps' reach throughout the world.

We cannot thank you enough.

About International Medical Corps

Founded in 1984, International Medical Corps is a leading first responder to natural disasters, conflict, and disease and is widely regarded as one of the most effective and efficient humanitarian organizations operating today.

International Medical Corps assists those in urgent need anywhere, anytime, no matter the conditions, providing lifesaving health care—often within hours of a sudden-onset crisis. Speed saves lives during the initial hours following a disaster. International Medical Corps' Emergency Response Teams deploy fast and begin their lifesaving work immediately, even in the most challenging environments.

International Medical Corps multiplies the impact of its work through training and by investing in people. International Medical Corps passes essential skills into local hands, preparing communities to better withstand adversity and be more resilient. Embedding these skills into the community lies at the heart of what International Medical Corps does: build self-reliance. It gives people hit by tragedy a sense of ownership in their recovery and the ability to shape their own future as they rebuild.

By providing healthcare through training, International Medical Corps goes far beyond simple direct delivery of relief, saving millions of lives while training local health care workers, who in turn go on to train others and care for their own communities. This multiplier effect is both high-impact and highly sustainable, helping the world's most vulnerable people recover, rebuild, and once again become self-reliant.

Since its founding, International Medical Corps has delivered lifesaving care and training to tens of millions of people in more than 75 countries.

INTERNATIONAL MEDICAL CORPS
TRAINING MANUAL MEDICAL DISCLAIMER

Knowledge and best practices in the medical field are constantly changing with new research and clinical experience and there may be reasonable differences in opinion among authorities. In addition, each situation has unique aspects that require independent consideration and judgment. Readers of this manual must always rely on their own experience, knowledge of the situation at hand, and judgment in evaluating and using any information in this manual, and are encouraged to consult and compare information from other sources. The treatments described and suggested in this manual are not absolute and universal recommendations. Further, any recommendations relating to drug selection and/or dosage in this manual may not be up-to-date or accurate. Readers are urged to check the most current information available to verify recommended dose or formula, the method and duration of administration, contraindications, or additional warnings or precautions.

International Medical Corps and the authors, editors, and other parties involved in the preparation of this manual are not responsible for errors or omissions or for any consequences from the application of the information in this manual and make no warranty, expressed or implied, with respect to the currency, completeness, availability, quality, or accuracy of the contents of the manual. To the fullest extent of the law, International Medical Corps and the authors, editors, and other parties involved in the preparation of this manual disclaim (and do not assume) any liability for any injury and/or damage to persons or property as a matter of products liability, negligence, or otherwise, or from any use or operations of any methods, products, instructions, or ideas contained in this manual.

Neither International Medical Corps nor the authors, editors, or other parties involved in the preparation of this manual recommend or endorse any specific tests, physicians, products, procedures, opinions, or other information that may be mentioned in this manual or otherwise obtained through a link or reference provided. Links and references are provided for informational and educational purposes only and do not constitute endorsement of any other sources, websites, manuals, materials, or other information. Information provided and opinions expressed by others do not necessarily represent the opinion of International Medical Corps. International Medical Corps expressly disclaims any and all liability resulting from reliance on such information or opinions.

Certain material in this manual is licensed to International Medical Corps by McGraw-Hill Education (the "McGraw-Hill Education Material"). McGraw-Hill Education makes no representations or warranties as to the accuracy of any information contained in the McGraw-Hill Education Material, including any warranties of merchantability or fitness for a particular purpose. In no event shall McGraw-Hill Education have any liability to any party for special, incidental, tort, or consequential damages arising out of or in connection with the McGraw-Hill Education Material, even if McGraw-Hill Education has been advised of the possibility of such damages.

ACKNOWLEDGEMENTS

The Editors wish to express appreciation and gratitude to the professionals and supporters who contributed to *The International Medical Corps Training Manual*.

Special thanks to Dawn Johnston, RN, Associate Editor, who worked tirelessly to coordinate the contributions to the *Manual* and review the compilation of a sizable amount of materials.

Warmest thanks to medical editor, Elizabeth Ross, whose dedication to accuracy and clarity created a much appreciated partnership with the *Manual* Editors. Medical Editor, Susan Duff, provided back-up in the massive undertaking.

The fine work of artists Jana Sliuzas, Laura Gajewski, Susan Gilbert, Susanna Dearwester, and Sarah Horton, who provided the original figures that illustrate the text, has been an important contribution.

Thanks to fact-checker Lynn Weber who worked closely with proof readers: Tricia Currie-Knight, Gary Hamel, Julia Loy, and Douglas NcNair.

Appreciation is due to Melissa Adams of The McGraw-Hill Companies, who has been both a supporter and advocate.

Thanks to Mary Daly for her dedication and commitment to this project and for keeping things moving with humor, patience, and persistence.

The International Medical Corps staff has been supportive and helpful. Special thanks to the IT Team, particularly Gabriel Valles, who have patiently provided the technical framework to support publication of the *Manual*.

This list would be incomplete if we did not thank both Marilynn Simon and Eleanor Hood who never wavered in their encouragement and enthusiasm.

About the Editors

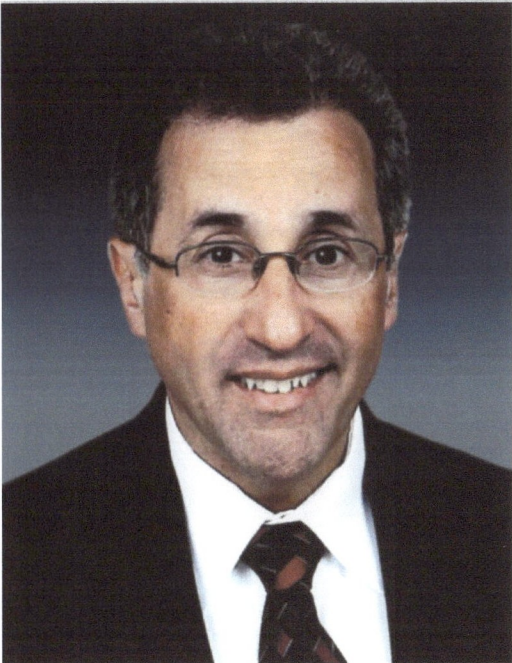

Dr. Robert Simon founded International Medical Corps in 1984 in response to the need for medical services and training inside war-torn Afghanistan. A renowned expert in Emergency Medicine, Dr. Simon is the author of numerous textbooks on orthopedic emergencies and surgical procedures, which are used as standards in Emergency Medicine throughout the United States. Dr. Simon is a professor in the Department of Emergency Medicine at Rush University, Stroger-Cook County Hospital in Chicago, Illinois. He is also former Bureau Chief of the Cook County Bureau of Health Services. He serves as Chairman of the Board of International Medical Corps.

Dr. Henry Hood is among the earliest International Medical Corps volunteers. An orthopedic surgeon in Lancaster, Ohio, Dr. Hood joined in 1985 to fulfill the organization's mission in the war in Afghanistan and in the refugee camps of Pakistan. In response to the need in Afghanistan, Dr. Hood solved a major medical problem of resource-poor environments, designing a traction system made out of wooden poles and rope that could be duplicated anywhere in the world. He has also volunteered in Somalia, Indonesia, and Haiti, among others. Dr. Hood has served as the Associate Board Chair of International Medical Corps since 1988.

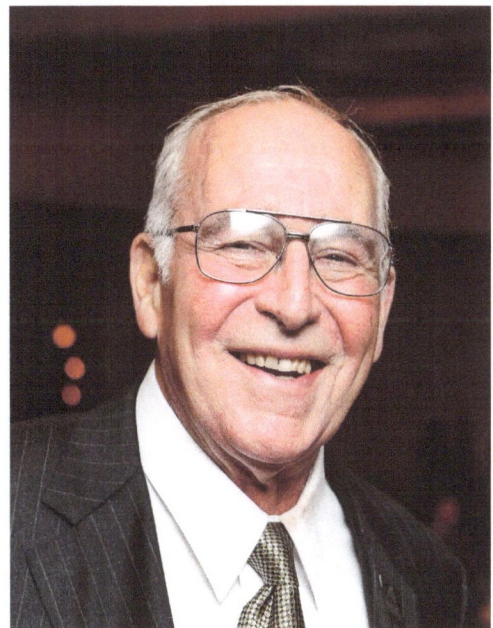

Contributors

Erica Ahlich

Paul Allegretti, DO, FACOEP

Amanda Amen

Evan Anderson

Alaina Antuma

Tiffany Aossey

Fatin Badran

Yusef A. Bazzy

Kara Bensley

Cameron Brenner

Caleb Cortes

Michael Joseph Cox

Heather Englert

Alan Gionetti

Kimberly Harden, MD

Danielle Hindi

Henry H. Hood, MD

Marian M. Houtman

Anwer Hussein, DO, FACOEP, FAAEM

Dawn Johnston

Stefanie Kosman

Adam Levine

Contributors (continued)

Ronald McLendon, MD, MPH

Holly McNally

Nathan Murphy-DuBay

Samantha Powers

Robert R. Simon, MD

Adam Simon

Timothy Simon

Rick Sly

Angela Taylor

Salvatore Termini

Kellie Turske

Karen Updike

Karla J. Wakim, DO

Andrea Wakim

Joe Walbridge

Justin Yax, DO, DTMH

Preface

This Manual seeks to provide a resource for the training of field medics and community health workers who would serve in under-resourced areas during conflicts or disasters. It targets those with a basic educational background and little or no prior medical education and, in conjunction with an intensive 4–8 week training program, will allow medics to diagnose and treat the most common 90% of illnesses and traumas. Based on a "Systems" approach (rather than symptom or specific disease orientation), the Manual covers basic anatomy and physiology and then focuses on the symptoms, physical findings, natural history, and differential diagnoses of the illnesses and injuries most likely to be encountered by health workers in the field. Treatment protocols are outlined, using those medications and materials likely to be found in under-resourced environments, including the generic medications of the WHO Essential Drugs List.

The purpose is to train field health workers quickly and give them the skills to treat the majority of wounded and ill in situations when whatever previous health care system there may have been is overwhelmed. Developing capacity and self-reliance by training persons from affected areas empowers individuals and communities — even those displaced from their homes — to regain control of their lives and destinies. This is the foundation of emergency humanitarian assistance.

This Manual, while a training manual, is also meant to be carried into the field as a ready reference for field health workers including trauma medics and community health workers as well as more highly trained medical personnel who may happen to find themselves practicing out of their areas of expertise. This could include national and international physicians, paraprofessionals, and nurses responding to a humanitarian emergency. This Manual does not intend to supersede local or national healthcare systems or protocols, but to provide an adjunct in an emergency when, as often happens, the perfect may be the enemy of the good.

Of necessity, much is omitted. Laboratory methods are covered in other manuals such as the excellent WHO publication. Medical and surgical procedures are left to other manuals such as *Tintinalli's Emergency Medical Manual* and James's *Field Guide to Urgent and Ambulatory Care Procedures* and the many institutional manuals covering the "how-to" of procedures.

Finally, public health considerations are not included in this field Manual; a companion manual describing public health and community interventions to target health promotion and prevention of injury and illness is planned.

Robert R. Simon MD and Henry H. Hood MD

February 2016

Note:

At the end of this volume you will find a list of Tables in this volume, more information about the editors, and the Master Table of Contents for all seventeen volumes of the Manual.

Contents

Chapter 1: Introduction to Cardiology   24

Anatomy and Physiology of the Heart — By Andrea Wakim   25

Approach to Chest Pain — By Ronald McLendon, MD, MPH   30

Introduction to Electrocardiograms (ECGs/EKGs) — By Dawn Johnston   41

Chapter 2: Cardiac Diseases and Disorders   49

Acute Coronary Syndrome — By Dawn Johnston   50

Angina Pectoris — By Robert R. Simon, MD   57

Acute Myocardial Infarction (Heart Attack) — By Robert R. Simon, MD   66

Pulmonary Edema — ByStefanie Kosman   78

Congestive Heart Failure — By Robert R. Simon, MD   86

Chapter 3: Arrhythmias   99

Sinus Node Dysfunction (SND) and Atrioventricular (AV) Block
   — By Marian M. Houtman   100

Bundle Branch Block — By Marian M. Houtman and Dawn Johnston   108

Supraventricular Tachycardia (SVT)
   — By Dawn Johnston and Marian M. Houtman   115

Multifocal Atrial Tachycardia (MAT) — By Dawn Johnston   122

Atrial Fibrillation — By Marian M. Houtman   127

Atrial Flutter — By Marian M. Houtman   138

Wolff–Parkinson–White Syndrome — By Marian M. Houtman   150

Premature Ventricular Contractions — By Marian M. Houtman   158

Ventricular Tachycardia — By Marian M. Houtman   165

Torsades de Pointes — By Marian M. Houtman 176

Ventricular Fibrillation — By Marian M. Houtman 185

Chapter 4: Venous Disease 192

Varicose Veins — By Marian M. Houtman 193

Superficial Venous Thrombosis — By Andrea Wakim 200

Chapter 5: Other Cardiovascular Conditions 204

Lymphedema — By Evan Anderson 205

Hypertension — By Michael J. Cox 207

Infective Endocarditis — By Evan Anderson 220

Abdominal Aortic Aneurysms and Acute Aortic Dissections
— By Evan Anderson 226

Peripheral Artery Disease — By Marian M. Houtman 232

Raynaud's Phenomenon — By Evan Anderson 238

Pericarditis — By Marian M. Houtman 242

Chapter 1:

Introduction to Cardiology

Anatomy and Physiology of the Heart
By Andrea Wakim

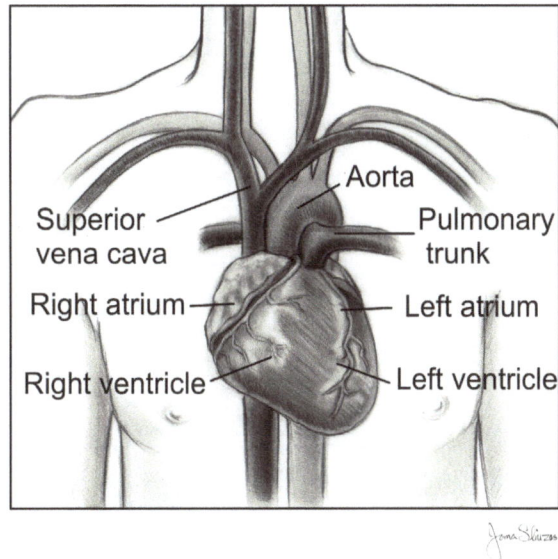

Figure 1.1 Anatomy of the Heart and Great Vessels.

- The heart is an organ made up of four chambers and various muscles.

- The chambers are the right and left atria, and the right and left ventricles.

- The atria collect blood and the ventricles pump blood.

- The right atrium and right ventricle deal with oxygen-poor blood, whereas the left atrium and left ventricle deal with oxygen-rich blood.

- Between each atrium and ventricle is a valve.

  ○ The valve between the right atrium and right ventricle is called the right atrioventricular valve or the tricuspid valve.

  ○ The valve between the left atrium and left ventricle is called the left atrioventricular valve or the bicuspid/mitral valve.

    ▶ When the ventricles contract, these valves close and block blood from leaking back into the atria.

      ▷ The valves are able to close because of chordae tendineae, thread-like fibers attached to the atrioventricular valves and papillary muscles on the inner walls of the ventricles.

      ▷ The contraction of the ventricles causes the papillary muscles to also contract, resulting in the chordae tendineae being pulled and shutting the atrioventricular valve to which they are attached.

○ Another set of valves, the semilunar valves—the aortic valve and the pulmonary valve—exist between the ventricles and adjoining major arteries.

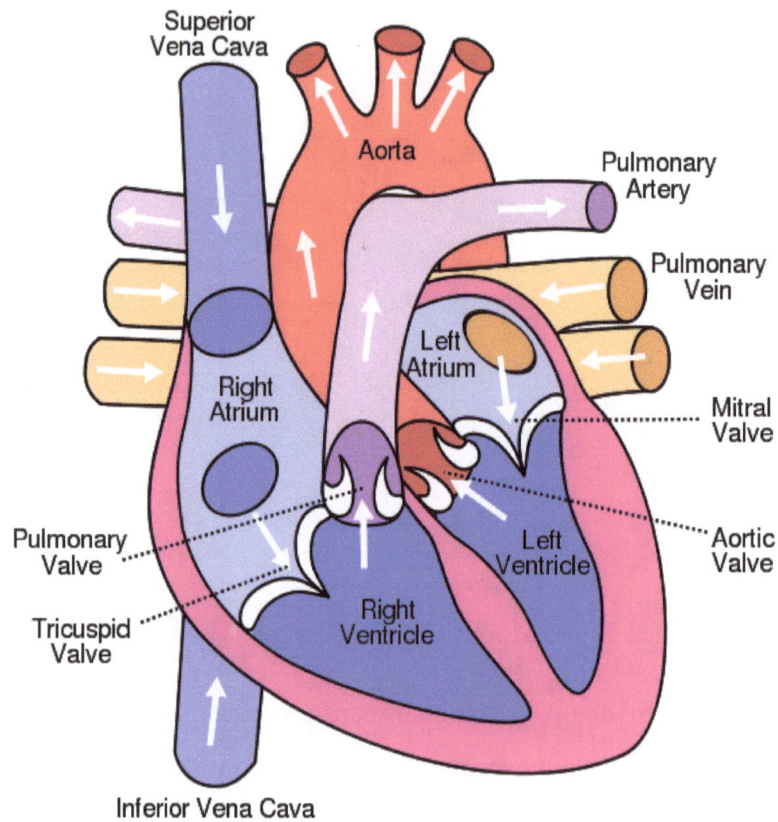

Figure 1.2 The Pulmonary and Systemic Circuits of the Heart.

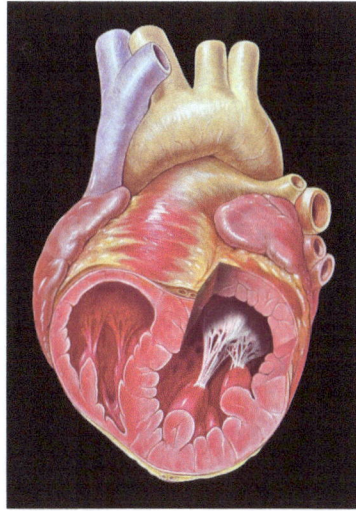

Figure 1.3 Cross-section of the Heart Showing the Papillary Muscles. These are attached to the fibrous chordae tendineae and the inner ventricular walls of the heart.

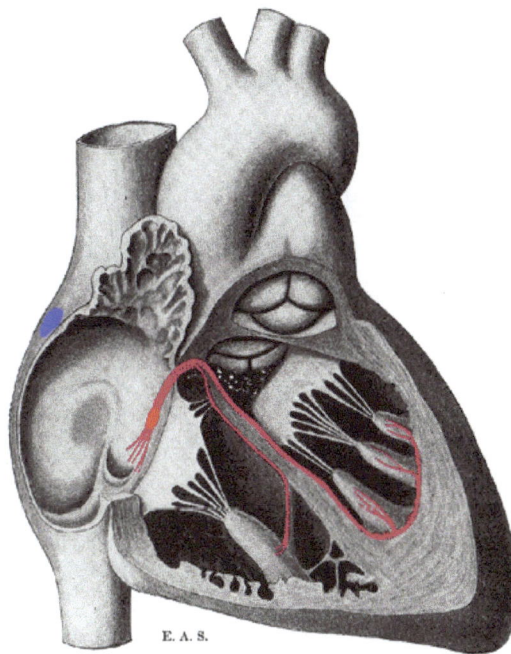

Figure 1.4 The Sinoatrial and Atrioventricular Nodes. The blue oval is the sinoatrial node. Through electrical signals controlled by the nervous system, electrical impulses travel to the atrioventricular node, the smaller red oval on the left half of the drawing. The bundle of His and Purkinje fibers extend into the inner ventricular walls and papillary muscles, stimulating the ventricles to contract.

- An artery is a blood vessel that carries blood away from the heart, as opposed to a vein, which is a blood vessel that returns blood to the heart.

- Two circuits of blood pass through the heart:
  - The pulmonary circuit
  - The systemic circuit
- The **pulmonary circuit** starts in the right atrium where blood passes through the right ventricle, pulmonary semilunar valve, and pulmonary artery, which branches in two and goes to each lung, where blood is oxygenated (enriched with oxygen).
  - In the capillaries (tiny blood vessels) of the lungs, oxygen-poor blood exchanges carbon dioxide for oxygen.
  - As a result, oxygen-rich blood leaves the lungs and returns to the left atrium of the heart through the pulmonary vein.
- The **systemic circuit** carries oxygen-rich blood via the pulmonary veins away from the lungs to the left atrium, then through the left ventricle, the aortic semilunar valve, the aorta, the upper and lower portions of the body, the superior and inferior vena cava, and finally back to the right atrium.
  - The aorta is the largest artery of the body, carrying blood to the upper and lower regions of the body.
  - The blood that returns through the superior and inferior vena cava to the right atrium is "oxygen-poor," meaning it lacks a significant amount of oxygen.
- Blood is pumped through the heart by the ventricles.
  - The coordination of the contraction of the ventricles is key.
  - This coordination is primarily controlled by the sinoatrial node, which lies in the right atrium.
    - ▶ The sinoatrial node is made up of a group of cells that sets the rate of contraction using electrical signals from nerve cells.
    - ▶ These electrical signals reach both atria, resulting in simultaneous contraction of the atria.
  - The signal is then delayed at the atrioventricular node to ensure that both atria have emptied entirely before the ventricles contract.
  - Then, muscle fibers known as the bundle of His and the Purkinje system relay the impulse to the bottom of the heart and back up the ventricular walls.
  - This mechanism triggers the strong and synchronized contractions of the ventricles that move blood out of the heart and into the arteries.
- When the heart pumps blood, or contracts, and then fills with blood again, or relaxes, it is known as the cardiac cycle. The cardiac cycle consists of two phases: diastole and systole.
  - In diastole, the heart is "relaxed" and blood flows into all four chambers of the heart because the atrioventricular valves are open and the semilunar valves are closed.

- ○ Systole is the contraction phase of the heart, beginning with a very short contraction of both atria that completely fills each ventricle with blood. Then, the ventricles contract:

  - ▶ The atrioventricular valves close and the semilunar valves open, allowing blood to be pumped into the aorta and pulmonary artery.

- ○ During the last part of systole, blood flows back into the atria, completing the cycle.

References

Anatomy of the Heart. NIH: National Heart, Lung and Blood Institute. www.nhlbi.nih.gov/health/health-topics/topics/hhw/anatomy.html

Healthwise Staff. Electrical System of the Heart. eMedicineHealth. www.emedicinehealth.com/electrical_system_of_the_heart-health/article_em.htm

How the Heart Works. WebMD. www.webmd.com/heart-disease/guide/how-heart-works?page=2

Figure 1.1 Anatomy of the Heart and the Great Vessels. Source: Jana Sliuzas, Medical illustrator.

Figure 1.2 The Pulmonary and Systemic Circuits of the Heart. Source: Eric Pierce / Wikimedia Commons / CC-BY-SA-3.0 / GNU Free Documentation License. Image at commons.wikimedia.org/wiki/File:Diagram_of_the_human_heart_(cropped).svg

Figure 1.3 Cross-section of the Heart Showing the Papillary Muscles. Source: Patrick J. Lynch / Wikimedia Commons / CC-BY-2.5 / Public Domain. Image at commons.wikimedia.org/wiki/File:Heart_short_axis_view_papillary.jpg

Figure 1.4 The Sinoatrial and Atrioventricular Nodes. Source: Henry Gray / Wikimedia Commons / Public Domain. Image at commons.wikimedia.org/wiki/File:Bundleofhis.png

Approach to Chest Pain
By Ronald McLendon, MD, MPH

Introduction

- Chest pain is one of the most common complaints patients have when seeking medical advice from health care professionals. This complaint can be frightening to an individual and should be thoroughly investigated.

- Many times, a patient's chest pain is not related to heart problems. This pain often involves other organ systems and can vary from mild to extreme in severity.

- Chest pain can be acute (sudden onset, short-lived) or chronic (persists for weeks or months) in nature. Regardless of its cause or severity, a complete work-up should be completed.

- The main causes of chest pain include:
  - Cardiovascular
  - Pulmonary
  - Musculoskeletal
  - Gastrointestinal
  - Emotional/mental

I. Review of Possible Causes

- **Cardiovascular**
  - Commonly located in one specific place in the body, or in several different locations, such as the middle of the chest, upper chest, back, arms (often the left arm), neck, and jaw.
  - May improve or worsen with rest or activity, and may be associated with other symptoms.
  - Could be described as crushing, sharp, dull, burning, pressure, or a feeling of tightness.
  - Pain can be intermittent (comes and goes) or constant, and may vary in intensity. It can also be associated with physical exertion or occur when the individual is at rest.
  - Chest pain associated with pulmonary vascular (affecting blood circulation in the lungs) origins can be similar to that of cardiac chest pain.

○ Pain may also be described as a tearing or ripping sensation, involving the chest, as well as the abdomen and back.

Table 1.1 Causes of Chest Pain

Cardiovascular	Pulmonary	Gastrointestinal	Musculoskeletal	Psychogenic (Originating in the Mind)
Angina (chest pain caused by reduced blood flow to the heart) Myocardial infarction (heart attack) Aortic dissection (a tear in the wall of the aorta) Valve disease Heart failure Endocarditis (inflammation of the endocardium, inner layer of the heart) Pericarditis (inflammation of the pericardium, the sac-like covering around the heart)	Asthma Bronchitis Pneumonia Pleuritis (inflammation of the lining of the lungs and chest) Pneumothorax (collapsed lung) Pulmonary embolism (blood clot blocking an artery in the lungs)	Esophageal rupture Esophageal motility disorder Reflux disease Peptic ulcer Biliary disease Pancreatitis	Muscle strain Costochondritis (inflammation of the cartilage that connects a rib to the breastbone) Virus (e.g., herpes zoster) Trauma	Anxiety Panic attack Hyperventilation Malingering (an exaggerated or pretended illness)

###

Radiation of pain into:
- The neck
- Left arm
- The back

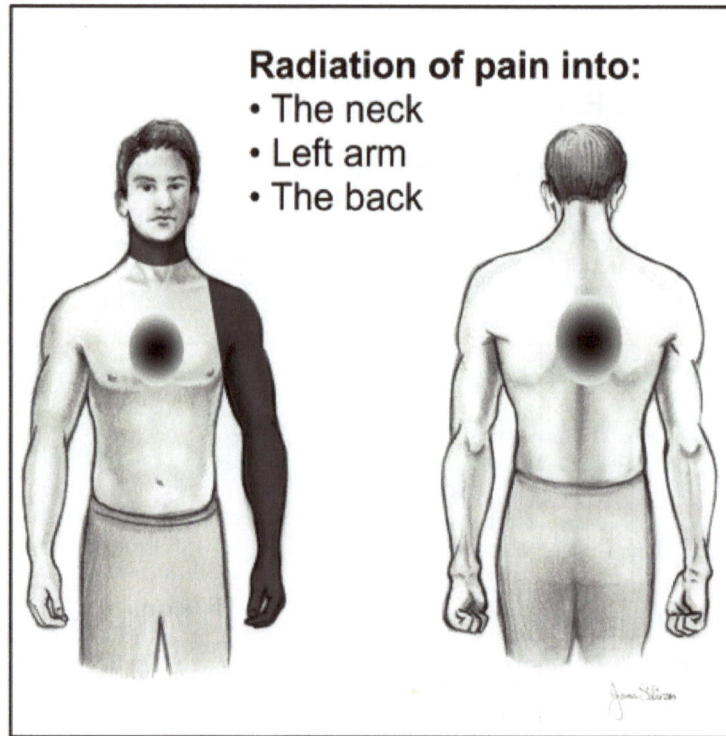

Figure 1.5 Radiation of Chest Pain.

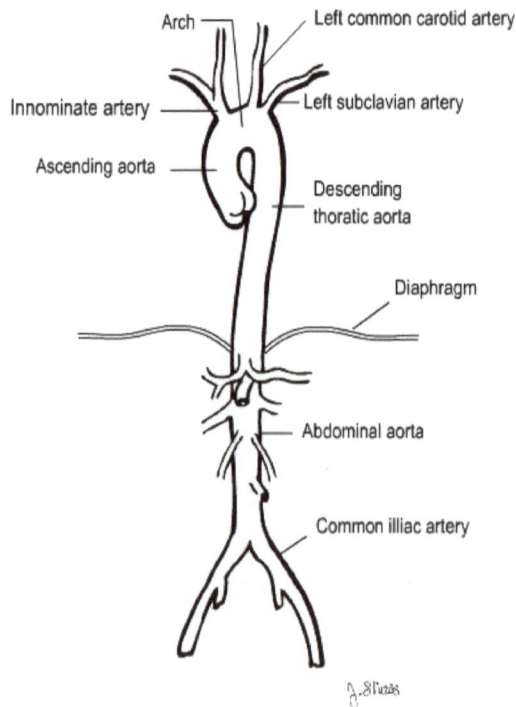

Figure 1.6 Anatomy of the Aorta.

● **Pulmonary**

- ○ Can occur in a specific location, or involve multiple areas
- ○ Intermittent or constant
- ○ Not necessarily felt in the center of chest
- ○ Sharp or achy in nature, with the pain lasting for several days
- ○ Can be localized to areas of the chest wall where the ribs cover the lungs, or felt in a location other than where the problem exists (this is known as referred pain).
- ○ Severity often worsens with inhalation or exhalation, as well as with coughing.
- ○ May be acute or chronic

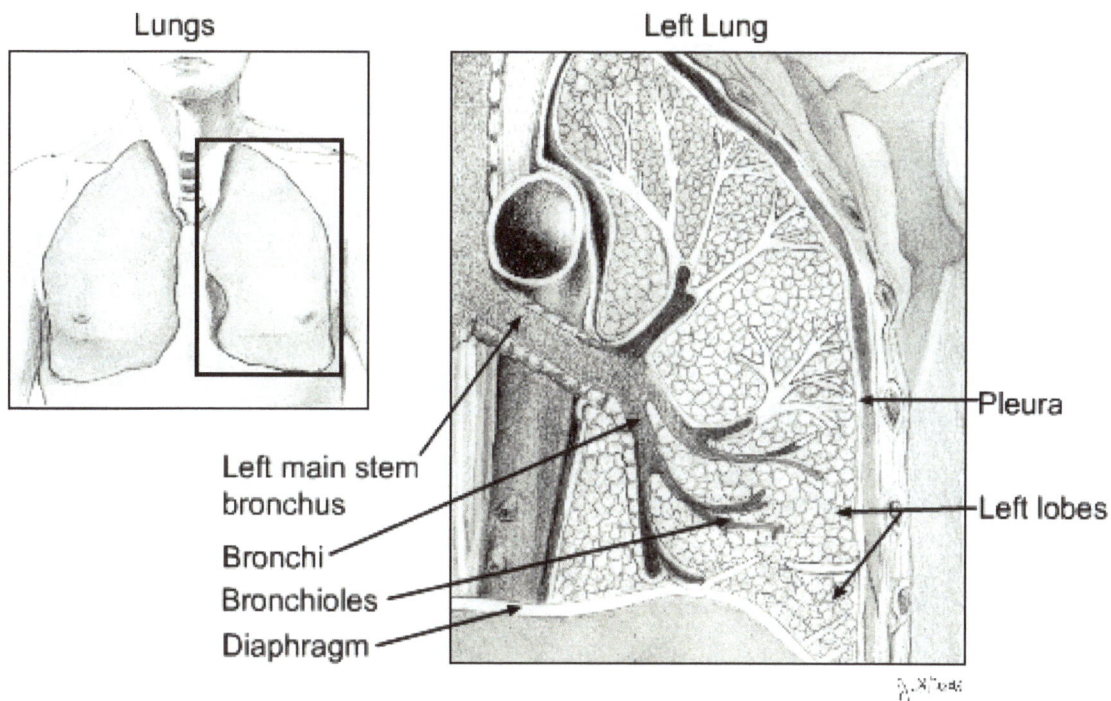

Figure 1.7 Pulmonary Structures that Commonly Cause Chest Pain.

● **Musculoskeletal**

- ○ Often slow in onset and persistent, lasting from a few hours to several weeks
- ○ Can involve skin, soft tissue, muscles, tendons, cartilage, and bones
- ○ Usually sharp and located in a specific area of the chest, such as the xiphoid process (the lowest portion of the sternum, or breastbone), mid-sternum and ribs; however, it can also be widespread and nonspecific
- ○ Can be related to body position, and worsened with arm movement, rotating, and deep breathing

    ○ Usually reproducible and painful to touch

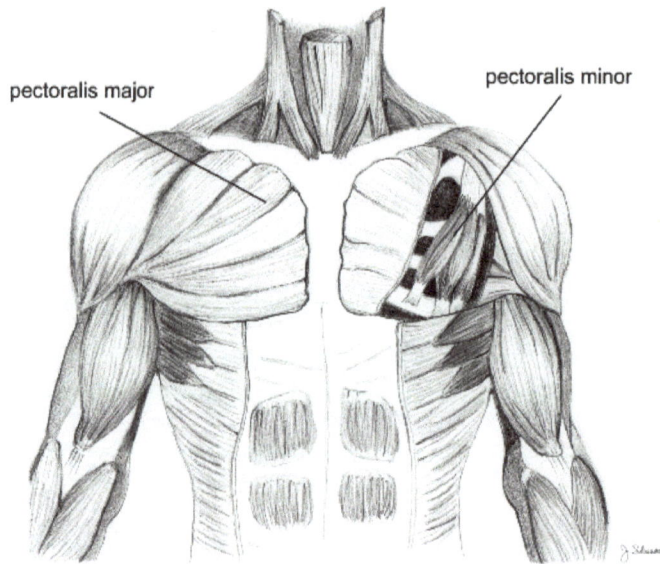

Figure 1.8 Musculoskeletal Anatomy of the Chest.

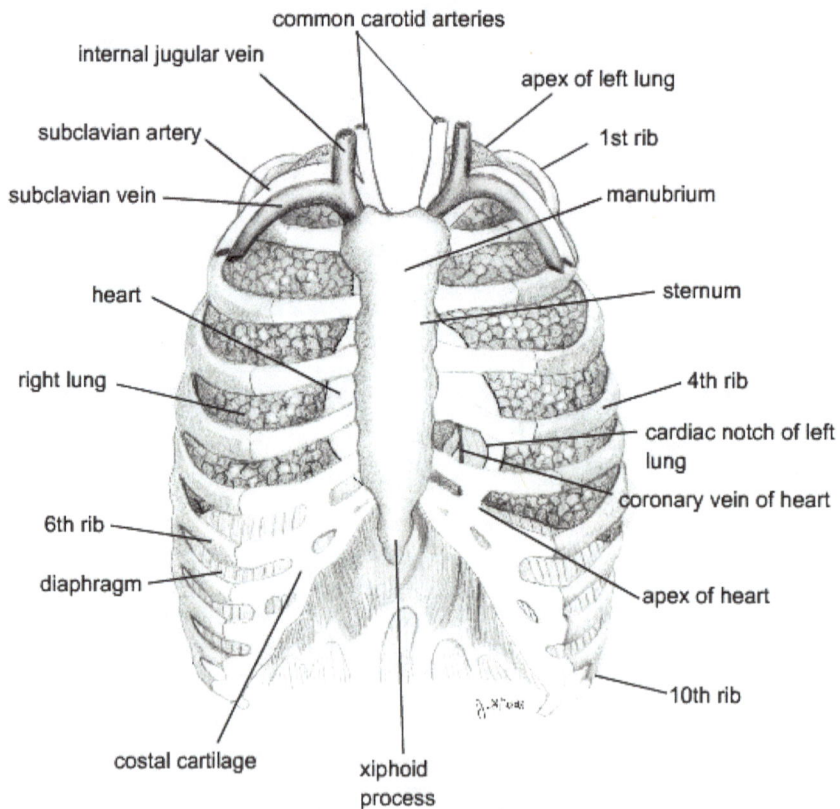

Figure 1.9 Anatomy of the Chest.

- **Gastrointestinal**
  - ○ Can be sharp, gnawing, or burning in nature, lasting from a few hours to several days
  - ○ Can be associated with eating spicy foods, drinking alcohol, consuming caffeine, or smoking
  - ○ A sour taste in the mouth may be experienced, as well as trouble swallowing.
  - ○ Often abdominal, but travels to the chest, causing pain in both areas simultaneously
  - ○ Can be related to body position and worsen when one lies flat

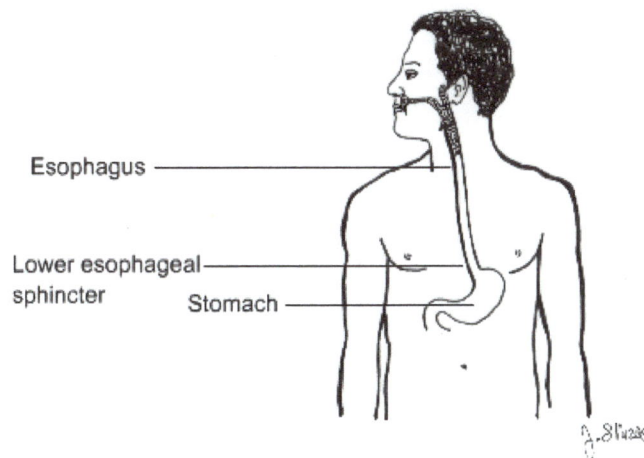

Figure 1.10 Digestive System Structures that Commonly Cause Chest Pain.

- **Psychogenic**
  - ○ Can be intense in nature, sometimes subjecting a patient to feelings of impending doom
  - ○ Associated with intense feelings of fear that occur without warning and usually for no apparent reason
  - ○ Can be sharp and abrupt, with chest wall soreness that may last from hours to days

II. Diagnostic Work-up

- A good history and physical exam are important in the evaluation for chest pain.
- Table 1.2 lists potentially life-threatening causes of chest pain that should be ruled out with a complete history, physical exam, and initial laboratory tests and studies, before considering other non-acute diagnoses.

Table 1.2
Signs and Symptoms of Potentially Life-Threatening Causes of Chest Pain

Diagnosis	Physical Exam: Common Findings	Common Descriptions of Pain	Associated Symptoms
Myocardial infarction (heart attack)	Hypertension (high blood pressure) or hypotension (low blood pressure) Tachycardia (abnormally fast heart rate) or bradycardia (abnormally slow heart rate) Elevated pressure in the jugular vein Heart murmur	Severely painful or mildly uncomfortable Exceeding 30 minutes Behind the sternum or in the upper middle abdomen Often brought on by exertion, heavy meals, or emotional distress, but may also be unprovoked Radiates to jaw, neck, arms or shoulder If there is a history of angina, new pain should differ in duration or severity, or may not respond to rest or nitroglycerin	Altered mental status Sweating Generalized weakness Light-headedness Nausea or vomiting Shortness of breath A tingling sensation in the hand(s) or fingers
Aortic dissection (a tear in the wall of the aorta)	Hypertension or hypotension Pulse deficits Heart murmur Neurologic deficits Paralysis	In chest, radiates to the back Sudden and maximal at onset Ripping, stabbing, or tearing If in the anterior chest, jaw, face, neck, or throat, it usually suggests ascending aorta If between the shoulder blades, in the back, abdomen or lower extremities, it usually suggests descending aorta	Absence of pulse in one or more extremity Weakness Stroke

Diagnosis	Physical Exam: Common Findings	Common Descriptions of Pain	Associated Symptoms
Pulmonary embolism (blood clot blocking an artery in the lungs) (Obtain patient's history, maintain a high level of clinical suspicion)	Tachypnea (rapid breathing) Rales (clicking or rattling lung sounds) Tachycardia Fever Lower extremity edema (swelling caused by excess fluid in the tissues) Heart murmur Cyanosis (bluish color to the skin or mucous membranes)	Symptoms and signs highly variable and nonspecific May be chest pain involving the lungs (inhalation) and may be very severe; however, there may be no chest pain History of recent surgery or immobility is often present	Shortness of breath Apprehension Cough Bloody cough Sweating Calf/thigh pain or swelling
Pneumothorax (collapsed lung)	Agitation Restlessness Tachycardia Tachypnea Hypotension Absent breath sounds on affected side	Sudden onset One side of the chest	Shortness of breath Low oxygen saturations
Esophageal rupture	Fever Tachycardia Tachypnea Hemoptysis (coughing up blood)	Frequently follows vomiting, but can also be associated with excessive coughing, heavy lifting, laughing, and seizures Pain usually located in the chest or abdomen, but location may vary	Nausea Vomiting Bloody vomit Sweating Difficulty swallowing Shortness of breath

Diagnosis	Physical Exam: Common Findings	Common Descriptions of Pain	Associated Symptoms
Pneumonia *See "Unit 16: Pulmonary" section of manual*	Fever Tachycardia Dyspnea (shortness of breath) with exertion Coarse lung sounds Productive cough	Pain with deep inspiration and sometimes with coughing	Dizziness sometimes associated with shortness of breath History of respiratory infection, often prolonged

- Perform an electrocardiogram (EKG/ECG).

  - Changes are usually seen in patients with ischemic chest pain (also called angina, or pain caused by reduced blood flow to the heart); however, a normal EKG does not rule out angina or myocardial infarction (heart attack).

  - If possible, have the patient's previous EKG available for comparison.

  - Review of serial EKGs is also important; these are usually ordered in conjunction with cardiac enzymes.

- Cardiac enzymes—enzymes that leak from damaged cardiac tissue—should be evaluated at regular intervals.

  - Myoglobin will be elevated within 3 hours of injury, peak in 4–9 hours, and return to baseline within 24 hours.

  - Creatine kinase myocardial band levels will be elevated within 4 hours of injury, peak within 12–24 hours, and return to baseline in 2–3 days.

  - Troponin-I will be elevated within 6 hours of injury, peak within 12 hours, and return to baseline in 3–4 days.

- Other laboratory tests

  - Basic metabolic panel to evaluate electrolyte abnormalities

  - Complete blood count to evaluate infection, high/low blood count, or platelet count

  - Urine analysis to evaluate renal function

  - D-dimer to rule out pulmonary embolism in patients with low pretest probability

  - Brain natriuretic peptide to measure severity of heart failure

- ○ Amylase to measure pancreatic activity (elevated during inflammation)
- ○ Lipase, similar to amylase, but more sensitive
- ○ Prothrombin time/international normalized ratio, and partial thromboplastin time to examine pathways involved in forming blood clots, and ability to clot blood
- ○ Fasting lipid panel to measure cholesterol
- ○ Liver enzymes
- ○ Urine drug screen to detect drugs in the system
- ○ Blood culture to rule out blood-borne infection
- ○ Sputum culture to rule out pulmonary infection
- ○ Arterial blood gas, used to determine the pH of the blood, the partial pressure of carbon dioxide and oxygen, and the bicarbonate level
- ● Studies and imaging
  - ○ Exercise stress test
    - ▶ Evaluate for evidence of decreased blood flow to the heart while the patient is active.
    - ▶ The patient walks or runs on a treadmill while being monitored by EKG.
    - ▶ Done after acute chest pain has resolved and patient is symptom-free
  - ○ Chest X-ray to evaluate the lungs, heart, ribs, sternum, and mediastinum.

III. Treatment

- ● The following should be done for every patient that presents with recent or ongoing chest pain:
  - ○ Assessment of airway, breathing, and circulation
  - ○ Introduction of supplemental oxygen
  - ○ Continuous cardiac monitoring
  - ○ Intravenous access established
  - ○ Assessment of vital signs
  - ○ Attach 12-lead EKG
  - ○ Order lab tests and imaging as directed by symptomology.
  - ○ Administer aspirin 325 mg by mouth, if no contraindications.
  - ○ Administer nitroglycerin under the tongue (***do not use*** if systolic blood pressure <90 mm Hg)
- ● See subsequent chapters in this unit for further treatment interventions for specific cardiac conditions.

References

Chest Pain. Mayo Clinic.
   www.mayoclinic.org/diseases-conditions/chest-pain/basics/definition/con-20030540

Chest Pain. MedicineNet.com. www.medicinenet.com/chest_pain/article.htm

Chest Pain. MedlinePlus. www.nlm.nih.gov/medlineplus/ency/article/003079.htm

Chest Problems. WebMD. www.webmd.com/heart-disease/tc/chest-pain-topic-overview

Desai, S. P. (2001). *Clinician's Guide to Diagnosis: A Practical Approach.* Hudson, OH: Lexi-Comp.

Figures 1.5–1.10 Source: Jana Sliuzas, Medical illustrator.

Introduction to Electrocardiograms (ECGs/EKGs)
By Dawn Johnston

Introduction

- The 12-lead electrocardiogram (called ECG or EKG) is a graphical means of interpreting the electrical activity of the heart.

- Correct interpretation of an ECG can help in the diagnosis of several conditions.

- Repetition is the best way to learn how to interpret an ECG.

I. Obtaining an ECG

- Apply the 4-lead ECG leads normally used to monitor a patient.

- Apply the precordial ("V") leads as shown in the diagram (Figure 1.11).

- Perform the 12-lead ECG as directed on the monitor, and print the results. (Note: a 12-lead ECG actually involves 10 electrodes, which together take 12 measurements.)

- Movement will affect the quality of the ECG. Ask the patient to breathe normally and avoid movement until the ECG is complete.

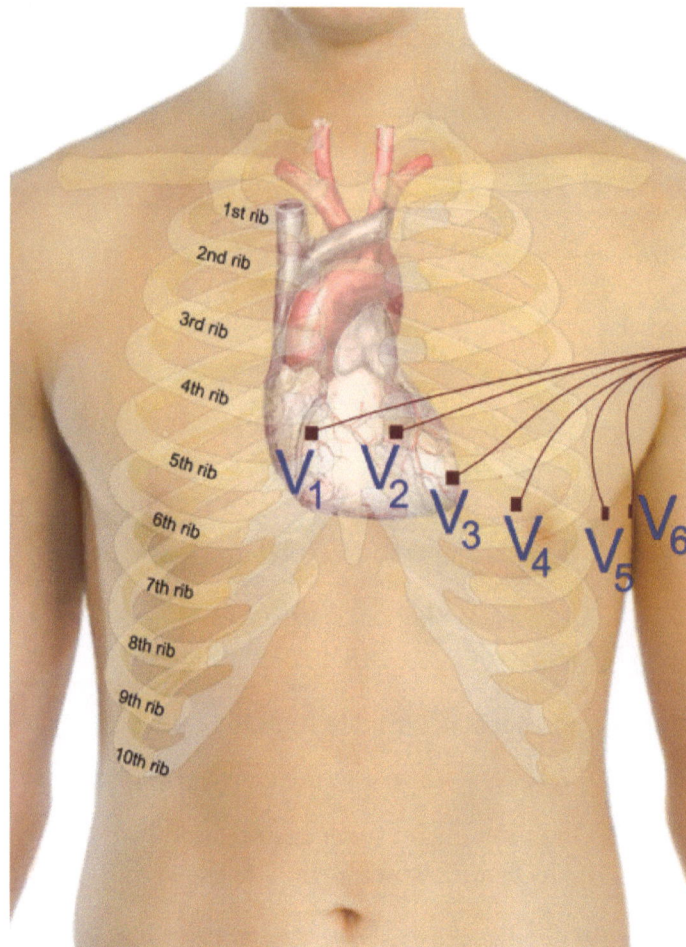

Figure 1.11 Placement of ECG Leads. An ECG is performed by the placement of six V-leads (as shown), in addition to four standard limb leads.

II. ECG Paper Measurements

- The graph paper for the 12-lead ECG enables the quantitative measurement of the electrical function of the heart.

  ○ Rate and rhythm are measured over time.

  ○ The height or "amplitude" of waveforms can be assessed for problems. For example:

    ▶ ST-segment elevation can be an indicator for acute myocardial infarction.

    ▶ Tall peaked T waves can indicate hyperkalemia (abnormally high level of potassium in the blood).

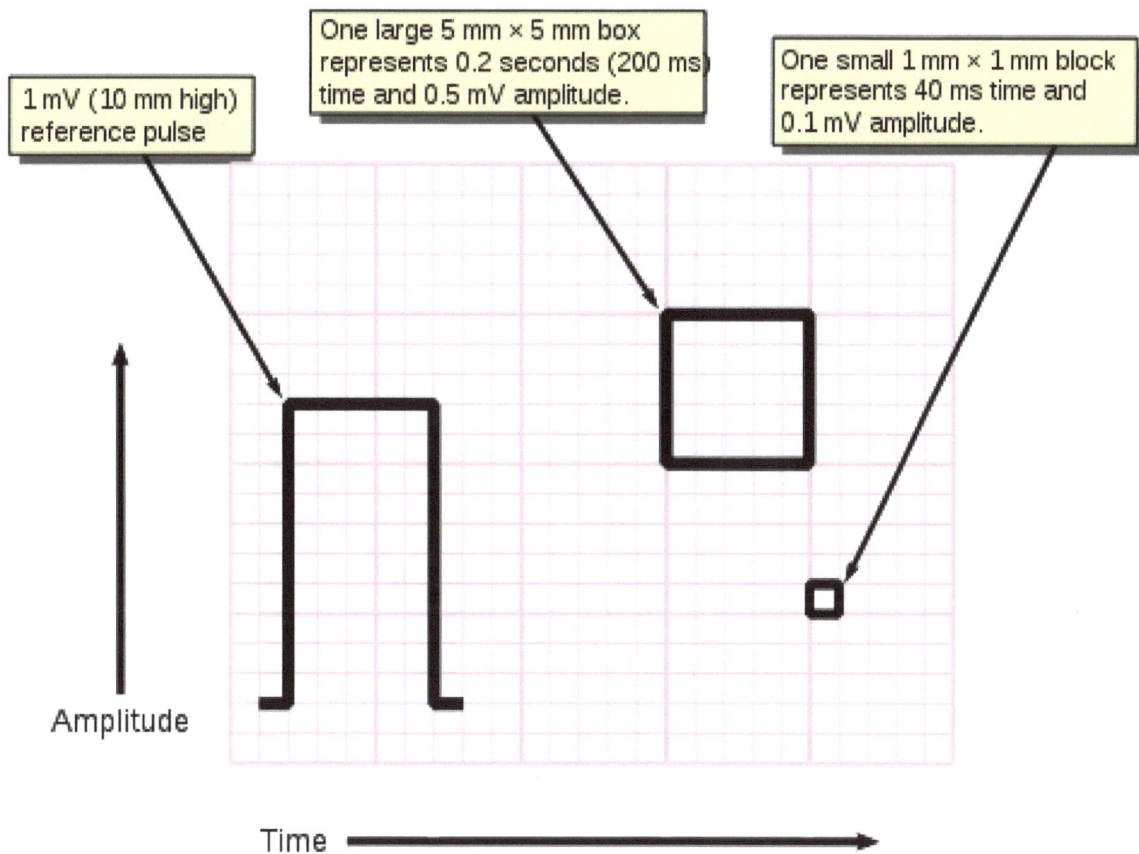

Figure 1.12 ECG Paper and Basic Measurements (enlarged to show detail).

- Each small 1x1 mm box represents:
  - ○ 0.04 seconds horizontally
  - ○ 0.1 mV amplitude vertically
- Each large 5x5 mm box represents:
  - ○ 0.2 seconds horizontally
  - ○ 0.5 mV amplitude vertically
- These standard measurements will help you assess whether an ECG is normal.

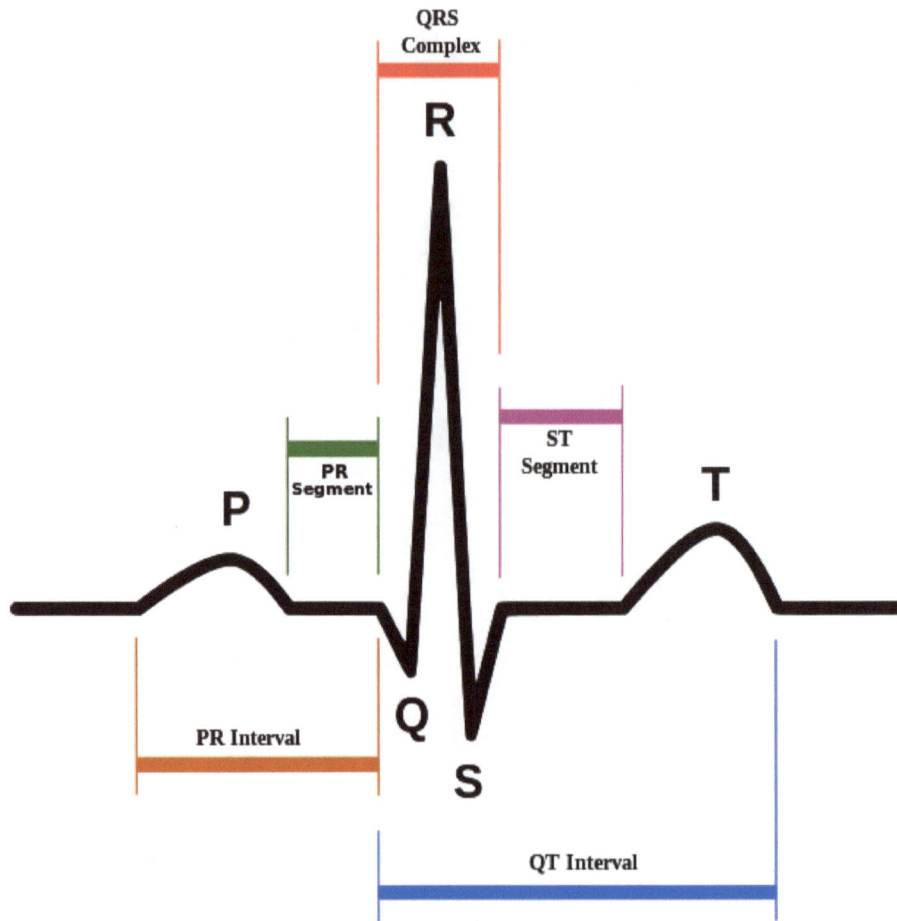

Figure 1.13 Tracing Generated by the Heart During Normal Contraction.

III. The QRS Complex

- A tracing generated by the heart during a normal contraction is shown in Figure 1.13.
- The isoelectric line is the initial horizontal line that heart deflections disturb.
  - This line is the "baseline" used to measure vertical height of some waves.
- Note that each deflection corresponds to an action in the heart.
  - Deflections can be positive (above the baseline).
  - Deflections can be negative (below the baseline).
- In normal sinus rhythm, the tracing deflections appear as follows:
  - P wave: electrical depolarization of atria
  - PR interval: atrial contraction
  - QRS complex: electrical depolarization of ventricles

    ○ ST segment: ventricles contract

    ○ T wave: repolarization of ventricles

● When the heartbeat tracing is recorded on the graph paper of an ECG (Figure 1.14), standardized measurements of the waves and intervals can be obtained.

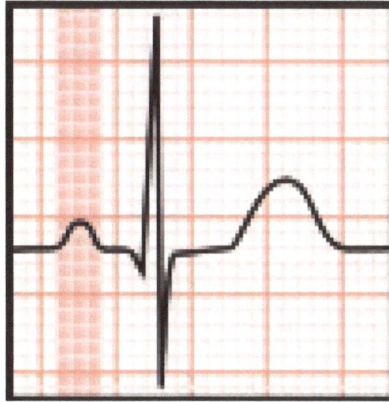

Figure 1.14 Intervals and Wave Forms on ECG. The intervals and waveforms of the heartbeat can be easily measured on ECG tracing paper.

● Normal values for key waves and intervals include:

    ○ PR interval: 0.20 seconds or less

    ○ QRS complex: 0.12 or less

    ○ QT segment: 0.40 or less

● Use these normal values to evaluate ECGs.

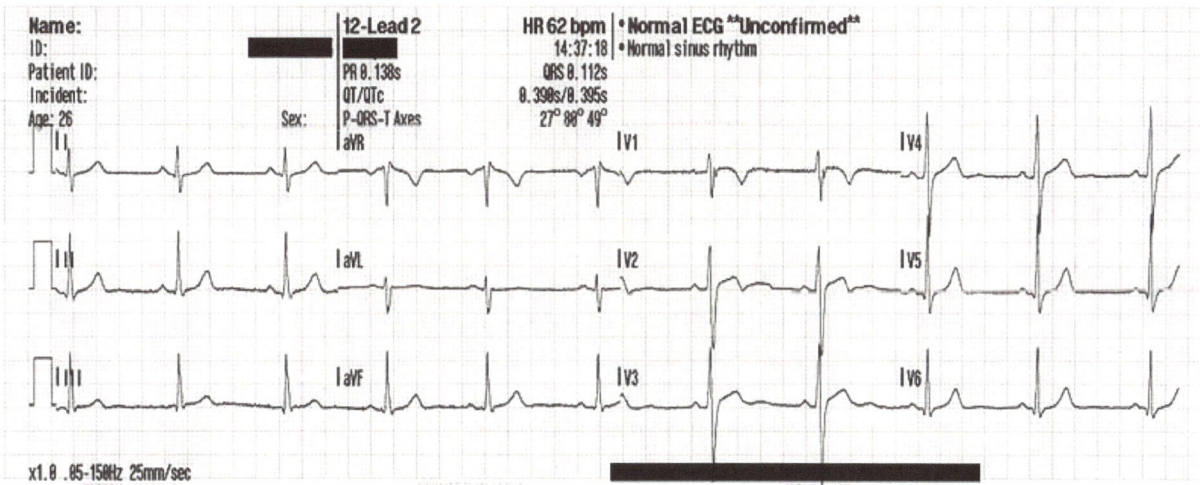

Figure 1.15 Normal ECG. Notable features include sinus rhythm, rate 62, no ST-elevation or ectopic beats (small changes in a heartbeat that is otherwise normal).

IV. Reading the ECG

- The ECG shows a "picture" of the heart from 12 different angles at the same time.

- Examining each lead on the ECG and considering the machine's interpretation will help diagnose whether a cardiac condition is present.

  ○ Each lead represents a location of the heart.

  ○ Some leads are redundant, and show pictures of the same area of the heart.

- Steps in interpretation:

  ○ Determine the rate and rhythm.

  ○ Assess the waves and intervals for abnormalities.

    ▶ Quantitative and qualitative measurements may be determined.

  ○ Correlate with patient condition.

    ▶ Consider the symptoms of the patient as you interpret the ECG.

V. ECG Example: ST-Elevation Myocardial Infarction (STEMI)

- When a patient presents with chest pain or other possible signs of heart attack (see the "Acute Myocardial Infarction [Heart Attack]" section in Chapter 2), perform an ECG.

- ST-elevation greater than 1 mm in two or more contiguous leads indicates acute myocardial infarction.

- The chart in Figure 1.16 resembles the location of leads on an ECG and explains which areas of the heart each lead represents. ST-elevation in two or more "same color" leads indicates STEMI.

I Lateral	aVR	V1 Septal	V4 Anterior
II Inferior	aVL Lateral	V2 Septal	V5 Lateral
III Inferior	aVF Inferior	V3 Anterior	V6 Lateral

Figure 1.16 Location of Leads.

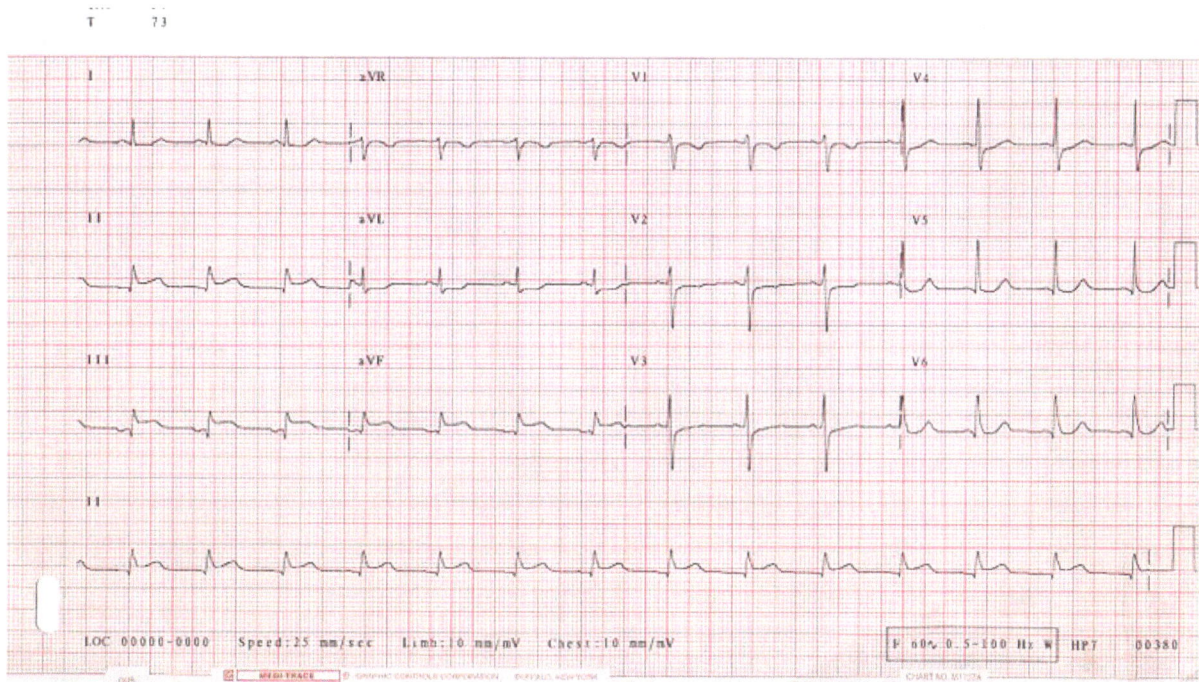

Figure 1.17 Sample ECG. This ECG shows sinus rhythm, rate 80s, with ST-elevation greater than 1 mm in leads II, III, and aVF, indicating an inferior wall myocardial infarction (heart attack). Reciprocal ST depression in other leads "mirrors" or confirms the STEMI diagnosis.

VI. Points for Further Study

- Repetition is essential when learning to read ECGs.

- Sinus tachycardia (abnormally fast heart rate) and sinus bradycardia (abnormally slow heart rate) are some of the most common abnormal ECGs.

- Always consider the patient's condition and context; for example, bradycardia can be a normal finding in an athlete with an exceptionally healthy heart.

- Acute ST-elevation myocardial infarction was explained here because it is a common emergency. See individual cardiology chapters for diagnosis-specific ECGs.

References

ECG Tutorial: Basic Concepts and Measurements. University of Michigan Health System. sitemaker.umich.edu/ecgtutorial/basic_concepts_and_measurements

Figure 1.11 Placement of ECG Leads. Source: Mikael Haggstrom / Wikimedia Commons / CC0-1.0. Image at commons.wikimedia.org/wiki/File:Precordial_leads_in_ECG.png

Figure 1.12 ECG Paper and Basic Measurements. Source: MoodyGroove / Wikimedia Commons / Public Domain. Image at en.wikipedia.org/wiki/File:ECG_Paper_v2.svg

Figure 1.13 Tracing Generated by the Heart During Normal Contraction. Source: Anthony Atkielski / Wikimedia Commons / Public Domain. Image at upload.wikimedia.org/wikipedia/commons/5/53/SinusRhythmLabels.png

Figure 1.14 Sample ECT. Source: Bron766 / Wikimedia Commons / CC-BY-SA-3.0. Image at commons.wikimedia.org/wiki/File:Normal_P_wave_(ECG).svg

Figure 1.15 Normal ECG. Notable features include sinus rhythm, rate 62, no ST-elevation or ectopic beats. Source: MoodyGroove / Wikimedia Commons / Public Domain. Image at commons.wikimedia.org/wiki/File:12leadECG.jpg

Figure 1.16 Location of Leads. Source: Cburnett / Wikimedia Commons / CC-BY-SA-3.0 / GNU Free Documentation License. Image at commons.wikimedia.org/wiki/File:Contiguous_leads.svg

Figure 1.17 Sample ECT. Source: Glenlarson / Wikimedia Commons / CC-BY-SA-3.0 / GNU Free Documentation License. Image at commons.wikimedia.org/wiki/File:ECG_001.jpg

Chapter 2:

Cardiac Diseases and Disorders

Acute Coronary Syndrome
By Dawn Johnston

Introduction

- Acute coronary syndrome is a broad term that describes sudden-onset cardiac events. These include:
  - ST-elevation myocardial infarction (STEMI)
  - Non-ST-elevation myocardial infarction (non-STEMI)
  - Unstable angina (USA)
- Acute coronary syndrome (ACS) is usually an indication of ruptured plaque and/or severe blockage of a coronary artery, causing blood-starved cardiac tissue to die.
- Any patient with chest pain requires immediate assessment for ACS and intervention, if necessary, to avoid, or prevent extension of, heart damage.

I. Pathophysiology

- The primary cause of ACS is atherosclerosis, the build-up of plaque (a fatty, waxy substance) in the coronary arteries.
  - When plaque is disturbed or ruptures, it creates an acute blockage.
- Sometimes stable coronary artery disease (CAD) can suddenly generate ACS due to a major stressor that increases the demand on the heart, such as:
  - Trauma, blood loss, anemia
  - Dehydration
  - Infection
  - Hypotension (low blood pressure)
  - Tachyarrhythmia (excessively rapid heartbeat accompanied by an irregular rhythm)
- Risk factors for the development of coronary artery disease that may lead to ACS include:
  - Smoking
  - Obesity
  - High cholesterol
  - Diabetes

○ High blood pressure

○ Poor diet with higher than recommended levels of fat, sugar, salt, and cholesterol

II. Clinical Signs and Symptoms

● The classic presentation of ACS is a patient clutching or holding his or her chest and grimacing, and complaining of chest pressure, squeezing, or "an elephant sitting on my chest."

○ Ask when symptoms started.

○ Use a 0 to 10 pain scale to track and treat pain.

● Symptoms may include:

○ Chest pain and/or pain in neck, jaw, shoulder, or either arm (usually the left)

○ Shortness of breath

○ Nausea

○ Cold, clammy skin

○ Palpitations

○ Heartburn

○ High or low blood pressure

○ Pulmonary edema (lung sounds: crackles or rales [clicking or rattling])

○ Jugular vein distention

○ Extra heart sounds

III. Diagnostic Work-up

● The ECG is the gold standard for diagnosis when ACS symptoms are present (see the "Acute Myocardial Infarction [Heart Attack]" section in Chapter 2).

○ Involve a cardiologist if at all possible and relay interpretation by phone; can make immediate transfer arrangements to a heart catheterization lab.

○ STEMI diagnosis:

▶ ST segment elevation at least 1 mm in two or more contiguous leads.

▶ ST segment depression in other leads helps confirm STEMI.

○ Non-STEMI/USA:

▶ No STEMI on ECG, but cardiac enzymes or physical presentation of patient indicate a major cardiac event.

● Assess vital signs; reassess every 15 minutes.

- Bloodwork
  - ○ Troponin levels every 6 hours three times (may have to transfer patient after the first one)
  - ○ Basic metabolic panel
  - ○ Complete blood count
  - ○ Myoglobin
  - ○ Creatine kinase isoenzyme MB (CK-MB)
- Imaging
  - ○ Chest X-ray is standard in the acute setting.
  - ○ Other imaging that may be useful:
    - ▶ Echocardiogram
    - ▶ Computed tomography (CT) scan
      - ▷ CT coronary angiography
      - ▷ CT coronary artery calcium scoring
    - ▶ Do not delay treatment for ACS when confirmed by ECG or lab work.

IV. Differential Diagnoses

Table 2.1 Differential Diagnoses for Acute Coronary Syndrome

Condition	Definition and Character	Signs and Studies
Cardiac		
Aortic dissection	A tear in the wall of the aorta. Sudden onset pain, stabbing, knife-like, radiating to back.	Asymmetric BP/pulses, widened mediastinum on chest X-ray
Myocarditis	Inflammation of the heart muscle, or myocardium. Sharp pain, worse with breathing.	Evaluate with echocardiogram
Pericarditis	Inflammation of the pericardium, the sac-like covering around the heart. Sharp pain worse with breathing, better when sitting forward, radiates to trapezius.	Diffuse ST-elevation on anterior leads of EKG with PR depressions in lead I; echocardiogram

Condition	Definition and Character	Signs and Studies
Tamponade	Pressure on the heart from buildup of blood or fluid in the space between the myocardium and pericardium. Significant shortness of breath, fatigue, low blood pressure (BP).	Distant heart sounds, increased jugular venous pressure, low BP, pulsus paradoxus (≥10 mm Hg drop in BP on inspiration)
Pulmonary		
Pulmonary embolus	Blood clot in large vessels of lungs, prevents oxygen-rich blood from reaching heart and other vital organs. Shortness of breath, sudden onset and worsening.	Rapid breathing, tachycardia, low oxygen in arterial blood, T-wave inversion in V1-V4 and ST-elevation in V1-V3.
Pneumonia	Lung infection, usually bacterial in origin. Mucus plugs small bronchioles/alveoli causing bacteria to grow and mucus to consolidate. Rapid breathing, fever, cough, pleuritic shortness of breath.	Maintain a high index of suspicion in elderly individuals, chronic smokers, COPD/asthma patients, and recently hospitalized, immune-suppressed and/or TB patients. Chest X-ray to look for consolidation, pleural effusion. Decreased breath sounds.
Tension pneumothorax	Presence of air in the space surrounding the lung(s). One-sided, sharp, pleuritic (affecting the membrane that surrounds the lungs), sudden pain	One-sided hyper-resonance, decreased breath sound. Chest X-ray to confirm.
Gastrointestinal		
Acid reflux	Movement of stomach acid into the esophagus. 5–60 minutes per episode.	Worse after eating food or lying down. Burning, usually in one spot, pain does not radiate, improves with food and antacid, normal EKG
Biliary (cholangitis, cholecystitis)	Bile stones block the biliary duct and cause inflammation and infection of gallbladder, common bile duct. More common in middle-aged women.	Continuous pain after eating. Episodic, after eating food, especially fatty foods. Positive Murphy's sign, elevated liver enzymes, bilirubin, amylase, lipase. Fever, if infected. Ultrasound of abdomen.
Esophageal (spasm, rupture)	5–60 minutes/episode, intense pain below sternum increased by swallowing.	Relief with nitroglycerin, normal EKG, evaluate with chest X-ray, barium swallow study.

Condition	Definition and Character	Signs and Studies
Pancreatitis	Inflammation of the pancreas. Continuous, sudden onset. Severe left upper quadrant pain with radiation to the back with nausea, vomiting.	History of alcohol drinking, trauma, scorpion bite. Elevated liver function tests, amylase, lipase, low bicarbonate.
Peptic/gastric ulcer	Prolonged period/episode, may be due to nonsteroidal anti-inflammatories (NSAIDs) or Helicobacter pylori bacteria. Usually experienced as a single "burning" spot; pain does not radiate.	Relief with food or antacid, normal EKG. Test for H. pylori antibody in serum, antigen in stool, ammonia in breath test.
Musculoskeletal		
Cervical disc disease	Caused by motion, lasts from seconds to hours.	Cervical X-rays
Costochondritis	Inflammation of the cartilage that connects a rib to the breastbone. Localized dull or sharp pain.	Tenderness to touch of chest
Rib fracture	Localized pain	Pain near sternum/rib on breathing
Herpes zoster	Viral disease commonly known as shingles. Intense one-sided pain.	Dermatomal rash (affecting only one side of the body in an area of skin where the sensory nerves are connected to a single spinal nerve root), sensory findings
Psychiatric		
Anxiety disorders, panic, hyperventilation	Tightness in the chest, shortness of breath.	Brought about by being in a particular situation (e.g., crowds)

###

V. Treatment

- The following is an overview of interventions for ACS; see the following sections on "Angina Pectoris" and "Acute Myocardial Infarction (Heart Attack)" for full treatment regimens.

- Treatment goals for ACS include:
  - Stabilizing the patient's pain, oxygenation (oxygen levels in the blood), and hemodynamics (blood flow/circulation)
  - Providing antithrombotic medication to prevent further blockage
  - Initiating early revascularization
    - ▶ Vessel is to be reopened within 90 minutes of first health care provider contact.
- Specific recommendations to achieve these goals include:
  - Initially, provide the following:
    - ▶ IV with normal saline; fluids as needed to keep blood pressure within normal limits.
    - ▶ Oxygen to keep saturations within patient's normal limits (ideally 94–99%)
    - ▶ Monitor patient for arrhythmias (abnormal heart rhythms) and treat according to advanced cardiovascular life support (ACLS) guidelines.
    - ▶ Give aspirin 162–325 mg; have patient chew for best absorption.
      - ▷ Only withhold if true aspirin allergy is present, meaning anaphylaxis (a severe, life-threatening allergic reaction).
    - ▶ Give nitroglycerin sublingual (under the tongue)
      - ▷ Avoid if hypotensive or if other signs of shock are present.
    - ▶ Provide pain control with morphine or fentanyl
      - ▷ Goal is to eliminate pain, which is an indicator for ischemia (insufficient supply of blood, usually due to a blocked artery)
      - ▷ Use with caution: narcotics can cause hypotension or loss of protective airway reflexes.
    - ▶ Clopidogrel 300–600 mg loading dose may be given.
    - ▶ Weight-based heparin bolus and infusion
    - ▶ Beta-blockers may be useful if patient is hypertensive (has high blood pressure) and has no contraindications.
  - Thrombolytics may offer a role if transfer times are extended.
    - ▶ Many contraindications and relative contraindications.
    - ▶ Relatively high risk of complications
      - ▷ Reperfusion arrhythmias are most common and may be deadly.
  - Transfer the patient to a facility capable of revascularization.
    - ▶ Heart catheterization lab to open/stent the occluded vessel.
    - ▶ Cardiac bypass surgery available in case the heart vessels are too diseased to be stented.

VI. Complications

- Ischemia
- Pulmonary edema
- Arrhythmias
- Rupture of cardiac structures
- Cardiac arrest

References

Coven, David L. Acute Coronary Syndrome. Medscape.
emedicine.medscape.com/article/1910735-overview

Sabatine, Marc S. (2008). *Pocket Medicine: The Massachusetts General Hospital Handbook of Internal Medicine* (Pocket Notebook Series) (3rd ed.). Philadelphia: Lippincott Williams & Wilkins.

Angina Pectoris
By Robert R. Simon, MD

Introduction

- Angina (angina pectoris) means "squeezing of chest."

- Angina is chest pain caused by a lack of blood oxygen to the heart muscle.

- Angina may be due to coronary artery disease (narrowing of the arteries due to hardened cholesterol fat).

- Stable angina is the most common type, occurring regularly, especially after exertion (e.g., climbing stairs), and lasting less than five minutes.

  ○ Patients with stable angina are taught how to avoid angina attacks and are often pre-scribed sublingual nitroglycerin as needed to manage these episodes.

- Unstable angina is less common and more serious. Pain occurs more frequently, lasts longer and may occur even at rest. It is often a sign of possible heart attack.

- All patients with angina are at risk of developing a heart attack (myocardial infarction).

I. Anatomical Points

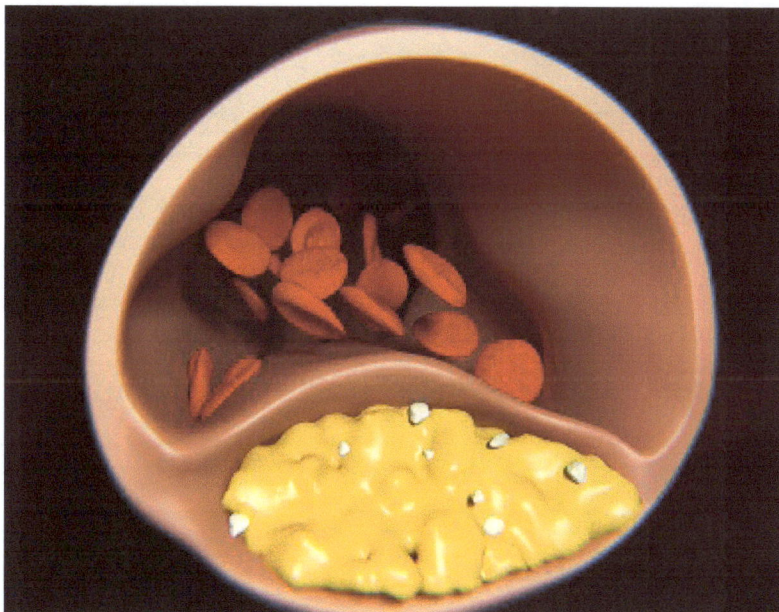

Figure 2.1 A Coronary Artery with Plaque Buildup. The plaque decreases blood flow.

II. Basic Physiology

- Angina occurs when the heart muscle is not getting enough blood oxygen.

- Narrowing of the arteries that deliver blood to the heart; blood flow may be slowed or blocked.

- Physical exertion, severe emotional stress, or heavy, fatty meals may cause angina.

- "Squeezing" chest pain may last one to 15 minutes per occurrence.

- Short attacks, from the lack of oxygen to the heart, may be reversible.

- Angina may be relieved by rest and medication.

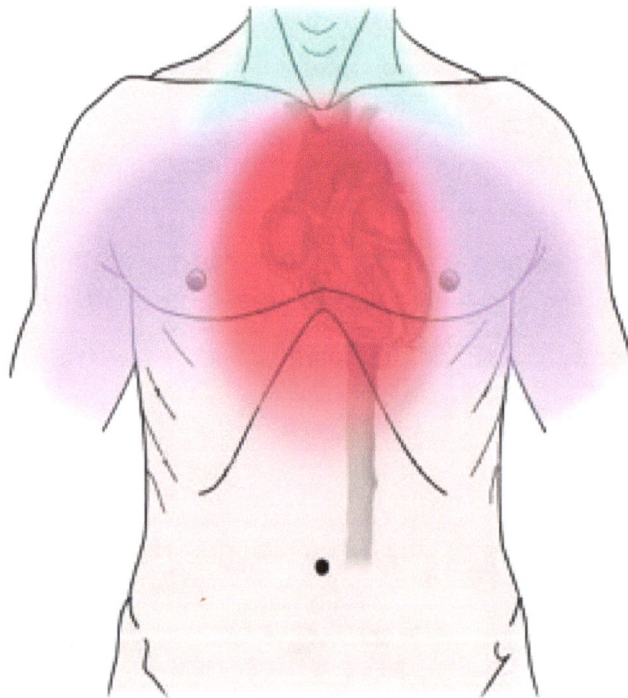

Figure 2.2 Chest Pain.

III. Clinical Signs and Symptoms

- Chest pressure
- Chest heaviness
- Chest tightening
- Chest squeezing
- Pain across chest, especially the center chest bone

- Pain may travel to neck, jaw, arms, back, or teeth

- Indigestion

- Weakness

- Sweating

- Upset stomach

- Cramping

- Shortness of breath

IV. Diagnostic Work-up

- An electrocardiogram (EKG/ECG) measures the heart muscle electrical activity and changes caused by lack of blood oxygen to the heart muscle. An EKG can show the following:

  - Insufficient blood flow to the heart (coronary heart disease)

  - A heart rate that is too slow, too fast, or irregular (arrhythmia)

  - Heart not pumping forcefully enough (heart failure)

  - Enlarged heart muscle (cardiomyopathy)

  - Defects in heart since birth (congenital heart defect)

  - Heart valve problems (heart valve disease)

  - Swelling or infection around the heart (pericarditis)

  - Rate and rhythm of the heartbeat can be traced and measured on a strip, which can help to determine underlying problems with the heart.

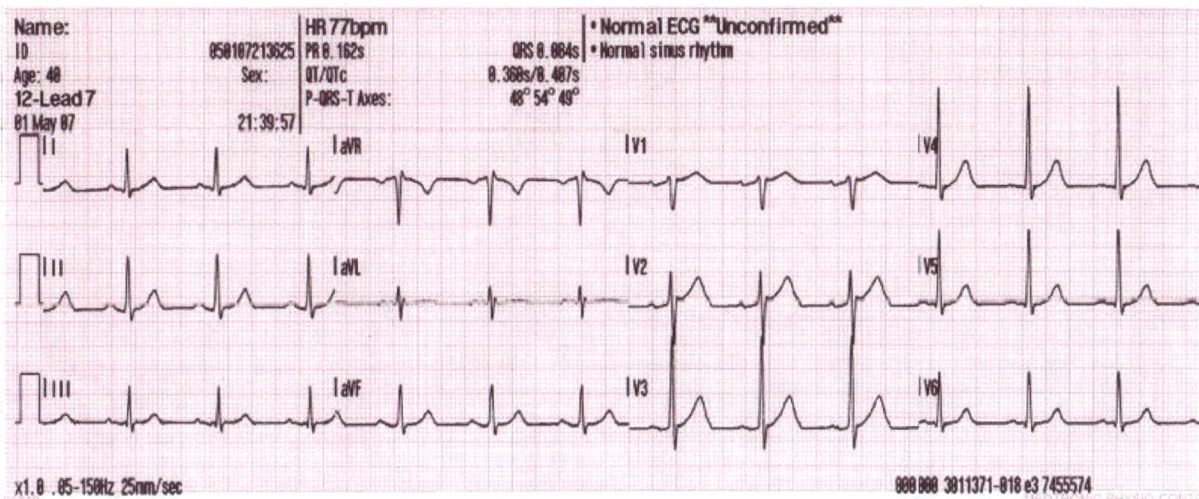

Figure 2.3 Normal Sinus Rhythm.

V. Differential Diagnoses

- Spasms of the esophagus (long food tube that connects mouth to stomach)

- Heartburn: burning sensation in the middle of chest (caused by acid reflux into the esophagus)

- Gall bladder attack: blockage causing pain in the upper abdomen, chest and/or back

- Inflammation of the chest wall, causing sharp chest pain which worsens with deep breathing and coughing

- Pneumonia: a bacterial or viral infection of the lungs causing fever and chest pain

- Pain from a rib fracture, muscle strain, or muscle spasm

- Anxiety and panic attacks may cause sharp or dull pain that can last from minutes to days, leading to rapid breathing, shortness of breath, and lightheadedness.

VI. Treatment

- After initial assessment of signs and symptoms and medical history, a patient with suspected angina will be given nitroglycerin sublingual (under the tongue) as a first approach to relieve pain.

- Monitoring of pain level and response to nitroglycerin can be measured and repeated every five minutes, up to three times, to treat angina.

- Other medications are recommended based on symptoms, and titrated (dosage adjusted to adequate levels) based on clinical response and lab work. Table 2.2 is followed by additional tables for lab work.

Table 2.2 Medication for Suspected Angina

Drug Name (Generic/Trade)	Adult Dosage	Action	Side Effects and Contraindications
Nitroglycerin, sublingual tablets (dissolve under tongue) (Nitro-Quick, Nitro-Tab, Nitro-Bid, Nitro-Stat, Nitro-Lingual spray)	0.3 mg 0.4 mg 0.6 mg	Immediate effect. Short acting, reduces spasms. Open blood vessels to the heart to bring in more blood/oxygen. May repeat every 5 minutes up to 3 times.	Lowers blood pressure (BP), flushing, dizziness, persistent throbbing headache, and increased heart rate. (Keep in dry container, avoid moisture.) Caution with decongestants, certain migraine, BP, and depression meds. Avoid alcohol and erectile dysfunction medications.

Drug Name (Generic/Trade)	Adult Dosage	Action	Side Effects and Contraindications
Transdermal patch (apply to skin) "(Nitro-Dur Nitro-Disc Transderm-Nitro)	0.1 mg/hour 0.2 mg/hour 0.3 mg/hour 0.4 mg/hour 0.6 mg/hour 0.8 mg/hour	For prevention of angina, coronary artery disease. Applied daily and long-term. Relaxes and widens blood vessels so the blood can flow more easily to the heart.	May lower BP, flushing, dizziness, headache, increased heart rate. Caution with decongestants, and certain migraine, BP, and depression medications. Avoid alcohol and erectile dysfunction meds.
Nitroglycerin ointment or cream (apply to chest) (Nitro-bid)	Put ½–2 inches of ointment onto a paper strip and apply onto skin and secure it. Apply every 4–6 hours.	For prevention of angina, coronary artery disease. Applied daily and long-term. Relaxes and widens blood vessels so the blood can flow easier to the heart.	Do not touch with fingers/hands. May lower BP and cause flushing, dizziness, headache, and increased heart rate. Caution with decongestants, and certain migraine, BP, and depression medications. Avoid alcohol and erectile dysfunction meds.
Nitroglycerin capsule/tablet (Nitrong, Nitro-Time)	2.5–9 mg 2–3 times daily 1–2 hours after meals	For prevention of angina, coronary artery disease. Applied daily and long-term. Relaxes and widens blood vessels so the blood can flow easier to the heart.	Lowers BP, may cause flushing, dizziness, persistent throbbing headache, increased heart rate. (Keep in dry container, avoid moisture.) Exercise caution with decongestants, and certain migraine, BP, and depression medications. Avoid alcohol, erectile dysfunction meds.
Isosorbide (Isordil Sorbitrate)	5–10 mg, chewable every 2–3 hours as needed. 2.5–10 mg sublingual every 2–3 hours as needed. 5–40 mg tablets every 8 hours.	For prevention or immediate treatment of angina. Opens blood vessels to the heart to bring in more blood/oxygen. Take on empty stomach to increase absorption.	Headaches and dizziness. Avoid alcohol. Caution for nursing mothers. May take with meals to reduce headaches. Tolerance may develop.

Drug Name (Generic/Trade)	Adult Dosage	Action	Side Effects and Contraindications
Aspirin	160–325 mg daily. Low dose if patient has stomach ulcers.	Antiplatelet. To help prevent blood clots. Thins the blood to limit damage to the heart.	Upset stomach or inflammation, abdominal pain, and bleeding. Should *not* use aspirin in: pregnant or nursing women; teenagers or children with fever, flu-like symptoms; patients with advanced liver or kidney disease; before surgery or invasive procedures.
Beta Blockers			
Atenolol (Tenormin)	50 mg daily for 1 week, then increase to 100–200 mg.	Decreases: heart rate, blood pressure, pump force of heart, heart's need for oxygen. Used for long-term/chronic treatment of angina, and particularly effective for exercise, stress-related angina.	May worsen asthma, chronic obstructive pulmonary disease (COPD). Excessive decrease in heart rate and blood pressure. May cause depression, excessive tiredness, a rise in "bad" cholesterol, increased shortness of breath from fluid retention (occurs in congestive heart failure). Monitor weight gain. Increases sensitivity to cold, skin eruptions. Do not stop medication abruptly. Do not use with MAO drugs. Avoid alcohol.
Metoprolol (Lopressor)	50 mg twice a day for one week, then 100–400 mg daily (increase dose at weekly intervals to desired effect)		
Propranolol (Inderal)	80–320 mg/day in 2–4 divided doses		
Propranolol, sustained release (Inderal SR)	80 mg SR/day, may increase to 160 mg/day		

###

Table 2.3 Cardiac Lab Tests
(Note: elevated cardiac enzymes may indicate damaged heart tissue)

Test	Patient Type	Lower Limit	Upper Limit	Unit
Creatine kinase (CK)	Male	24, 38, 60	174, 320	U/L or ng/mL
		0.42	1.5	µkat/L
	Female	24, 38, 96	140, 200	U/L or ng/mL
		0.17	1.17	µkat/L
CK-MB		0	3, 3.8, 5	ng/mL or mcg/L
Myoglobin	Female	1	66	ng/mL or mcg/L
	Male	17	106	

####

Table 2.4 Cutoffs and Ranges for Troponin Types, 12 Hours After Onset of Pain

Test	Lower Limit	Upper Limit	Unit	Comments
Troponin-I		0.2	ng/mL or mcg/L	Upper limit of normal
	0.2	1.0	ng/mL or mcg/L	Acute coronary syndrome
	0.4	2.0	ng/mL or mcg/L	Moderately increased
	1.0, 1.5	n/a	ng/mL or mcg/L	Myocardial infarction likely

###

Table 2.5 Other Significant Blood Tests

Test	Patient Type	Lower Limit	Upper Limit	Unit	Therapeutic Target
Triglycerides	10–39 years	54	110	mg/dL	<100 mg/dL or 1.1 mmol/L
		0.61	1.2	mmol/L	
	40–59 years	70	150	mg/dL	
		0.77	1.7	mmol/L	
	>60 years	80	150	mg/dL	
		0.9	1.7	mmol/L	
Total cholesterol		3.0, 3.6	5.0, 6.5	mmol/L	<3.9
		120, 140	200, 250	mg/dL	<150
HDL cholesterol	Female	1.0, 1.2, 1.3	2.2	mmol/L	>1.0 or 1.6 mmol/L >40 or 60 mg/dL
		40, 50	86	mg/dL	
	Male	0.9	2.0	mmol/L	
		35	80	mg/dL	
LDL cholesterol (Not valid when triglycerides >5.0 mmol/L)		2.0, 2.4	3.0, 3.4	mmol/L	<2.5
		80, 94	120, 130	mg/dL	<100
LDL/HDL quotient		n/a	5	(unitless)	

###

- Lifestyle changes:
  - Stop smoking
  - Healthy diet to avoid high fats and sugars
  - Control high blood pressure
  - Regular exercise
  - Reduce stress
- The patient should report chest pain that occurs more often, lasts longer, or is more painful, as well as shortness of breath that occurs even while resting, dizziness, or spreading of pain to other areas.
- The patient should return to be re-checked if he or she is placed on medication to treat and control angina.

Special thanks to contributor Diane M. Garcez.

References

Angina. WebMD. www.webmd.com/heart-disease/tc/angina-topic-overview

EKG. NIH: National Heart, Lung, and Blood Institute. www.nhlbi.nih.gov/health/health-topics/topics/ekg

Reference Ranges for Blood Tests. Wikipedia. en.wikipedia.org/wiki/Reference_ranges_for_blood_tests#Cardiac_tests

Spratto, G.R., and Woods, A.L. (2005). *PDR Nurse's Drug Handbook*. New York: Delmar Learning.

Wedro, Benjamin. Angina. MedicineNet.com. www.medicinenet.com/angina_symptoms/article.htm

Figure 2.1 A Coronary Artery with Plaque Buildup. Source: U.S. Centers for Disease Control and Prevention; Division for Heart Disease and Stroke Prevention, Coronary Artery Disease (CAD) / Public Domain. Image at www.cdc.gov/heartdisease/coronary_ad.htm

Figure 2.2 Chest Pain. Source: Ian Furst. File:Angina pectoris.png. CC-BY-SA-3.0. Image at commons.wikimedia.org/wiki/File:Angina_pectoris.png

Figure 2.3 Normal Sinus Rhythm. Source: Glenlarson / Wikimedia Commons / Public Domain. Image at commons.wikimedia.org/wiki/File:12_lead_generated_sinus_rhythm-2.JPG

Acute Myocardial Infarction (Heart Attack)
By Robert R. Simon, MD

Introduction

- Myocardial infarction (MI) is a "heart attack" that happens when a blood clot blocks the blood flow through the coronary arteries to the heart muscle.

- Heart attacks may be due to coronary artery disease, a narrowing of the arteries from hardened cholesterol fat.

- A heart attack causes death of tissue, and permanent damage to the muscles of the heart.

- The extent of this damage depends on the size of the clot, the area deprived of blood, and how much time passes between when the attack occurs and when treatment is started.

- MI that shows STEMI on ECG requires the clogged vessel to be opened or "reperfused" either by percutaneous coronary intervention (PCI) at a heart catheterization lab, or with thrombolytic medications.

- MI with non-STEMI signs on ECG may be treated medically, but their condition may ultimately require PCI, as well.

I. Basic Physiology

- Heart disease occurs when the arteries that supply blood to the heart become narrow.

- Narrowing of the arteries causes blood flow to the heart to be slowed down or blocked.

- Angina (chest pain) occurs when the heart muscle is not getting enough blood oxygen.

- The blockage (plaque) is made up mostly of cholesterol (fat), which builds up and hardens, eventually breaking off to form floating clots.

- A heart attack occurs when this plaque blocks an artery, stopping blood flow/oxygen to an area of the heart, which dies.

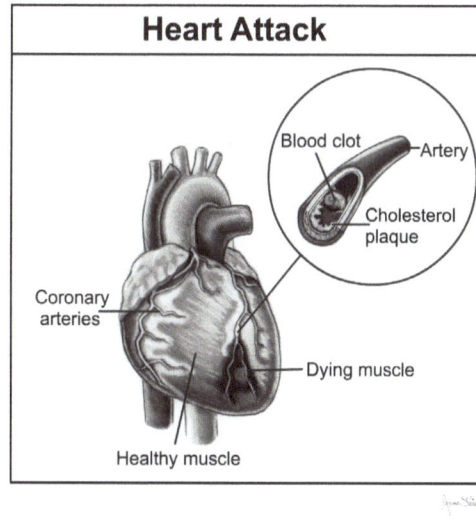

Figure 2.4 Blockage of an Artery Due to Plaque Buildup. This blockage causes a decrease in blood flow.

II. Clinical Signs and Symptoms

- Discomfort, pressure, heaviness, or pain in the chest
- Pain moving into the back, jaw, left arm
- "Heartburn," indigestion, fullness, throat tightness
- Sweating, upset stomach, vomiting
- Dizziness, weakness, shortness of breath, nervousness
- Rapid or irregular heartbeat (arrhythmias)
- Symptoms can last 30 minutes or longer.
- Can start as mild discomfort and progress to severe pain, or occur as sudden, severe pain
- Some people, most commonly women and patients with diabetes, experience no symptoms during a heart attack ("silent" MI).
- Women may describe symptoms as:
  - Neck and shoulder pain
  - Abdominal pain
  - Sick to stomach (nausea)
  - Vomiting
  - Extremely tired (fatigued)
  - "Hard time breathing" (shortness of breath)

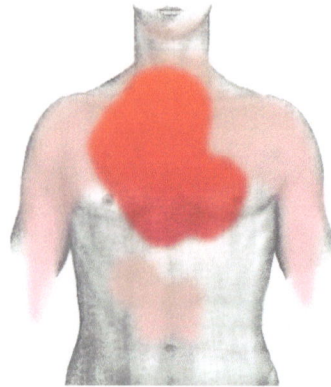

Figure 2.5 Typical Areas of Chest Pain (red) and Radiating Pain (pink) to the Neck, Jaw, Either Arm, or Epigastric Region.

III. Diagnostic Work-up

- Electrocardiogram (ECG/EKG)
  - ○ Measures the heart's electrical activity, and can detect:
    - ▶ Insufficient blood flow to heart (coronary heart disease)
    - ▶ A heart rate that is too slow, too fast, or irregular (arrhythmia)
    - ▶ Heart not pumping forcefully enough (heart failure)
    - ▶ Enlarged heart muscle (cardiomyopathy)
    - ▶ Defects in heart since birth (congenital heart defect)
    - ▶ Heart valve problems (heart valve disease)
    - ▶ Swelling or infection around the heart (pericarditis)
  - ○ The heartbeat's rate and rhythm can be traced and measured on a strip, and can help determine underlying problems with the heart.

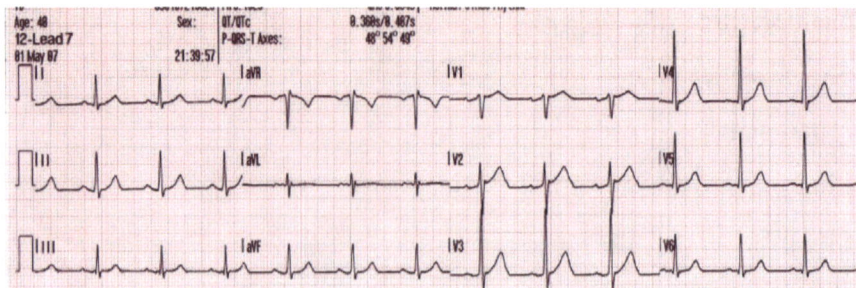

Figure 2.6 Normal Sinus Rhythm: 60–100 Beats per Minute.

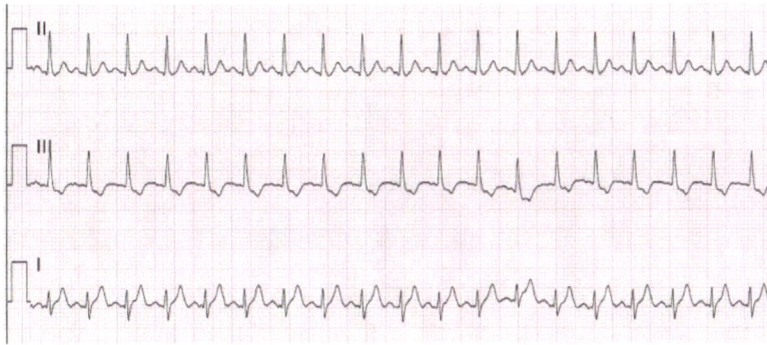

Figure 2.7 Sinus Tachycardia. The heart is beating too fast: over 100 beats per minute.

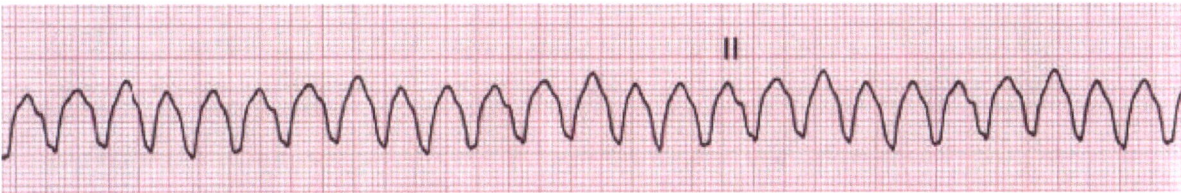

Figure 2.8 Abnormal Pattern—Ventricular Tachycardia.

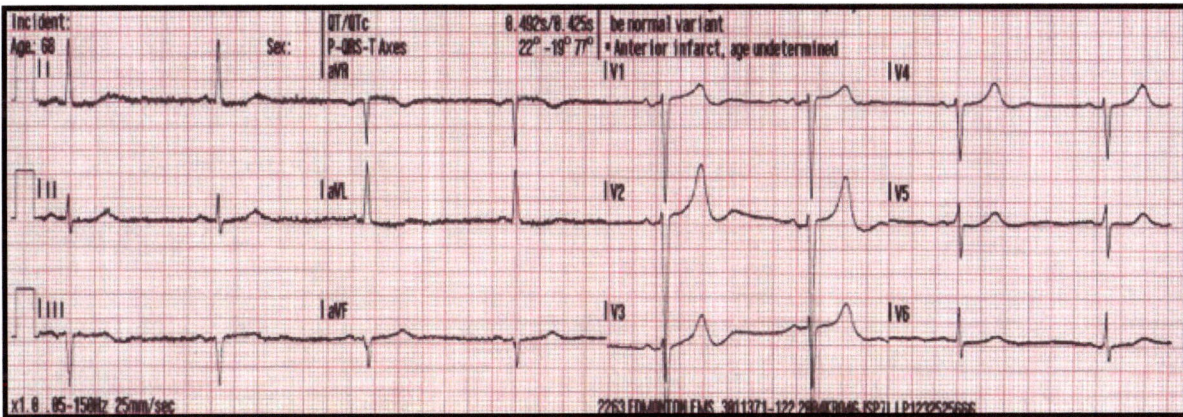

Figure 2.9 Sinus Bradycardia. Heart is beating too slowly: less than 60 beats per minute.

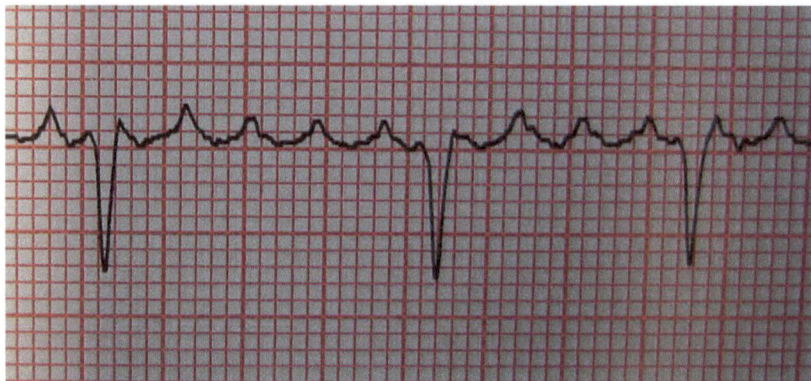

Figure 2.10 Atrial Flutter. Saw-tooth appearance; not pumping well, and usually 250–300 beats per minute.

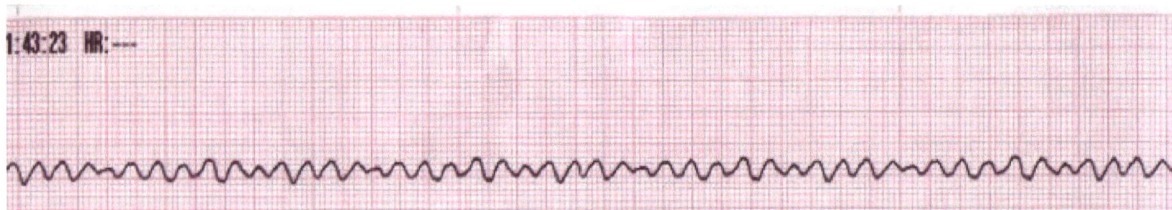

Figure 2.11 Ventricular Fibrillation. Irregular, random, incomplete beats.

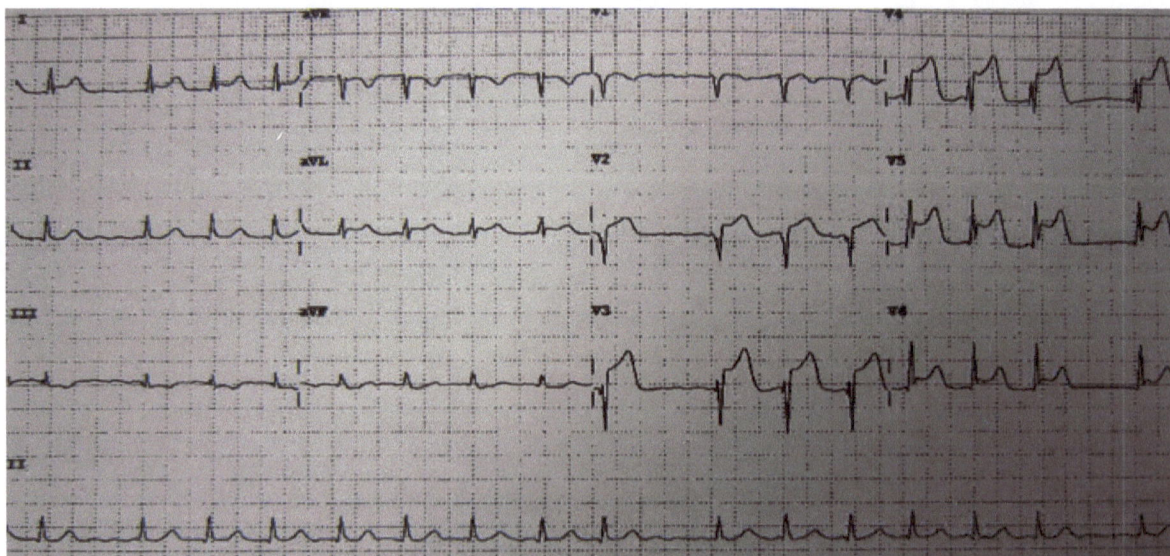

Figure 2.12 Anterior Wall MI.

Table 2.6 Laboratory Tests
(cardiac enzymes may increase due to damaged heart tissue)

Blood Test	Range (Units/L)	Comments
Creatine kinase (CK) male	38–174	Muscle damage
Creatine kinase (CK) female	96–140	
CK-MB	0–5	Amount of damage
Myoglobin/male	17–106	Injury to heart
Myoglobin/female	1–66	
Troponin-I	<0.2	Measures cardiac muscle damage
Troponin-I	0.2–1.0	Heart disease
Troponin-I	1.0–.5	Heart attack likely
Troponin-T	<0.02	Normal
Troponin-T	0.02–0.10	Heart disease
Troponin-T	>0.10	Heart attack likely
Triglycerides	70–150 mg/dL	Goal: <100 mg/dL
Total cholesterol	100–199 mg/dL	Goal: <150 mg/dL
HDL cholesterol	40–86 mg/dL	Female
HDL cholesterol	35–80 mg/dL	Male
LDL cholesterol	80–130 mg/dL	Goal: <100 mg/dL

- Chest X-ray
  - Examine the chest for the following signs that the heart's pumping ability is failing:
    - Fluid buildup in the lungs
    - Enlarged heart

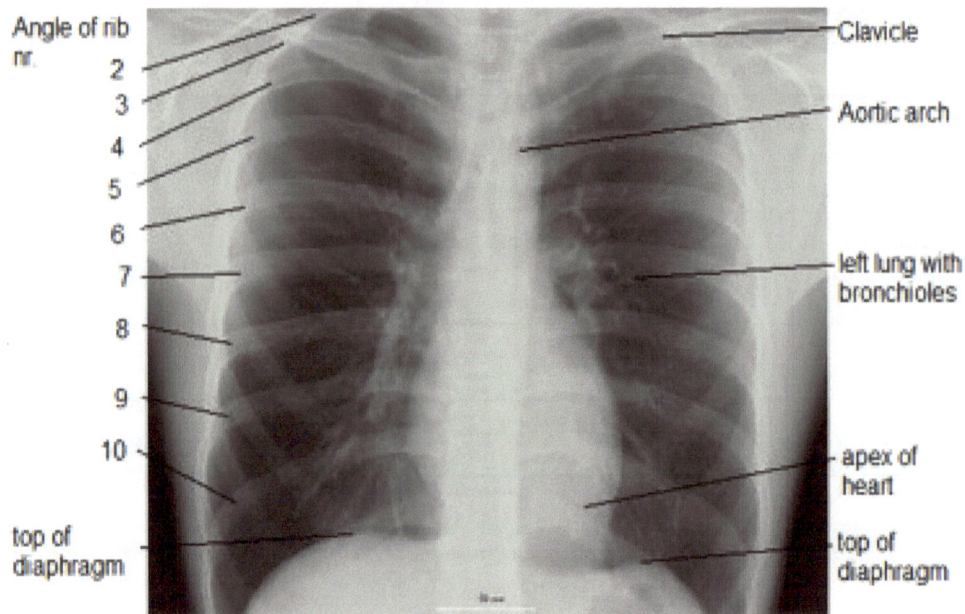

Figure 2.13 Chest X-ray.

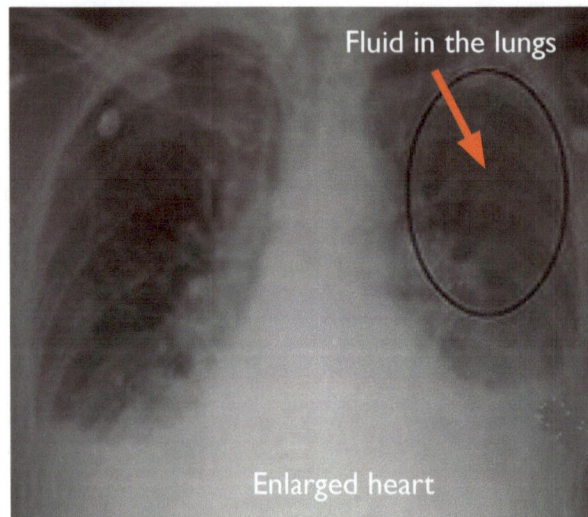

Figure 2.14 Chest X-ray with Enlarged Heart and Fluid Accumulation (appears as gray areas in the lungs).

IV. Differential Diagnoses

- Spasms of the esophagus (long food tube that connects mouth to stomach)
- Heartburn (burning sensation in the middle of chest caused by esophageal reflux)
- Gallbladder attack: blockage causing pain in the upper abdomen, chest and/or back

- Inflammation of the chest wall; sharp chest pain that worsens with deep breaths, coughing

- Pneumonia: a bacterial or viral infection of the lungs causing fever and chest pain

- Pain from a rib fracture, muscle strain, or spasm

- Anxiety and panic attacks may cause sharp or dull pain that can last minutes to days, leading to rapid breathing, shortness of breath, and lightheadedness.

V. Treatment

- Patients with STEMI confirmed by ECG or non-STEMI confirmed by positive cardiac enzymes should be transferred to a facility with cardiology services capable of percutaneous heart catheterization and open-heart surgery.

- In an *alert* (awake and attentive) patient with suspected angina or heart attack:

  - Nitroglycerin sublingual (under tongue) administered first to relieve the chest pain.

  - Monitoring of pain level and response to nitroglycerin can be measured, and administration of medication can be repeated every five minutes, up to three times, to treat chest pain.

  - Intravenous (IV) fluids by needle, into a large vein, usually in the arm

  - Normal saline or Lactated Ringer's at 100 mL/hour (approximately 4 drops/minute)

  - Oxygen by nasal cannula (tube placed outside of nose). Start at 2L airflow.

  - Check blood pressure, pulse rate and rhythm, respirations (how many breaths per minute; typical rate for adults is 12–20) and oxygen level (pulse oximetry, goal 92–100%).

  - Continual care; medications are prescribed after a heart attack to:

    - Prevent future blood clots/blockages

    - Help the heart work better and with less effort

    - Prevent narrowing of the arteries (lower cholesterol/fats)

    - Treat irregular heartbeats

    - Lower blood pressure and control chest pain

    - Treat other complications from heart failure/damage

Table 2.7 Drugs Used for MI: Dosing, Action, and Side Effects/Contraindications

Drug Name	Dose Adult	Action	Side Effects and Contraindications
Nitroglycerin, sublingual tablets *(under tongue to dissolve)* (Nitro-Quick, Nitro-Tab, Nitro-Bid, Nitro-Stat, Nitro-Lingual spray)	*For chest pain.* 0.3 mg 0.4 mg 0.6 mg	Immediate effect. Short acting, reduces spasms. Open blood vessels to the heart to bring in more blood/oxygen. May repeat every 5 minutes up to 3 times	Lowers blood pressure (BP), may cause flushing, dizziness, persistent throbbing headache, increased heart rate. Keep in dry container, avoid moisture. Caution with decongestants, and certain migraine, BP, and depression medications. Avoid alcohol and erectile dysfunction medications.
Transdermal Patch *(apply to skin)* (Nitro-Dur Nitro-Disc Transderm-Nitro)	0.1 mg/hour 0.2 mg/hour 0.3 mg/hour 0.4 mg/hour 0.6 mg/hour 0.8 mg/hour	For prevention of angina, coronary artery disease. Applied daily and long-term. Relaxes and widens blood vessels so the blood can flow more easily to the heart.	May lower BP, cause flushing, dizziness, headache, and increased heart rate. Caution with decongestants, and certain migraine, BP, and depression medications. Avoid alcohol and erectile dysfunction medications.
Nitroglycerin ointment or cream *(apply to chest)* (Nitro-bid)	Place ½–2 inches of ointment onto a paper strip and apply it onto skin and secure it. Apply every 4–6 hours.	For prevention of angina, coronary artery disease. Applied daily and long-term. Relaxes and widens blood vessels so the blood can flow more easily to the heart.	Do not touch ointment/cream with fingers/hands. May lower BP, cause flushing, dizziness, headache, and increased heart rate. Caution with decongestants, and certain migraine, BP, and depression medications. Avoid alcohol and erectile dysfunction medications.
Nitroglycerin capsule/tablet (Nitrong Nitro-Time)	2.5–9 mg 2–3 times daily 1–2 hours after meals	For prevention of angina, coronary artery disease. Applied daily and long-term. Relaxes and widens blood vessels so the blood can flow more easily to the heart.	Lowers BP, may cause flushing, dizziness, persistent throbbing headache, increased heart rate. Keep in dry container, avoid moisture. Caution with decongestants, and certain migraine, BP, and depression medications. Avoid alcohol, erectile dysfunction medications.

Drug Name	Dose Adult	Action	Side Effects and Contraindications
Isosorbide (Isordil Sorbitrate)	5–10 mg, chewable every 2–3 hours as needed. 2.5–10 mg under tongue every 2–3 hours as needed. 5–40 mg tablets every 8 hours	For prevention or immediate treatment of angina. Opens blood vessels to the heart to bring in more blood/oxygen. Take on empty stomach to increase absorption.	Headache, dizziness. Avoid alcohol. Caution in lactating women. May take with meals to reduce headaches. Tolerance may develop.
Aspirin	Patient to chew tablet with onset of chest pain. 325 mg, then 160–325 mg daily	Antiplatelet. To help prevent blood clots. Thinning of blood to limit damage to the heart.	If patient has stomach ulcers, use low dose. Side effects include upset stomach, abdominal pain, inflammation of the stomach, bleeding. Do not use: pregnant or nursing, teenagers or children with fever or flu-like symptoms, patients with advanced liver or kidney disease, before surgery or invasive procedures.
Beta Blockers			
Atenolol (Tenormin)	*For high blood pressure.* 50 mg daily for 1 week, then increase to 100–200 mg.	Decreases: heart rate, blood pressure, pump force of heart, heart's need for oxygen For long-term treatment of angina; chronic angina For treatment of exercise or stress induced angina	May worsen asthma, COPD. Excessive decrease in HR, BP. Depression. Excessive tiredness. Cold sensitivity. Skin eruptions. Increased cholesterol, shortness of breath from fluid retention (from congestive heart failure). Monitor weight gain. Do not stop medication abruptly or use with MAO drugs. Avoid alcohol.
Metoprolol (Lopressor)	50 mg twice a day for one week, then 100–400 mg daily (increase dose at weekly intervals to desired effect)		

Drug Name	Dose Adult	Action	Side Effects and Contraindications
Propranolol (Inderal)	80–320 mg/day in 2–4 divided doses	Decreases: heart rate, blood pressure, pump force of heart, heart's need for oxygen	May worsen asthma, COPD. Excessive decrease in HR, BP. Depression. Excessive tiredness. Cold sensitivity. Skin eruptions. Increased cholesterol, shortness of breath from fluid retention (from congestive heart failure).
Propranolol, sustained release (Inderal SR)	80 mg SR/day, may increase to 160 mg/day	For long-term treatment of angina; chronic angina For treatment of exercise or stress induced angina	Monitor weight gain. Do not stop medication abruptly or use with MAO drugs. Avoid alcohol.

###

Special thanks to contributor Diane M. Garcez.

References

Angina. MedicineNet.com. www.medicinenet.com/angina

Angina. WebMD. www.webmd.com/heart-disease/tc/angina-topic-overview

Automated External Defibrillators. eMedicineHealth. www.emedicinehealth.com/automated_external_defibrillators_aed/page5_em.htm#

EKG. NIH: National Heart, Lung, and Blood Institute. www.nhlbi.nih.gov/health/health-topics/topics/ekg

How to Handle Heart Emergencies. WebMD. www.webmd.com/heart-disease/handle-cardiac-emergencies

Lead Generated Sinus Rhythm. WikiMedia. commons.wikimedia.org/wiki/File:12_lead_generated_sinus_rhythm.jpg

Reference Ranges for Blood Tests: Cardiac Tests. Wikimedia Commons / CC-BY-SA. en.wikipedia.org/wiki/Reference_ranges_for_blood_tests#Cardiac_tests

Figure 2.4 Blockage of an Artery Due to Plaque Buildup. Source: Jana Sliuzas, Medical illustrator.

Figure 2.5 Typical Areas of Chest Pain (red) and Radiating Pain (pink) to the Neck, Jaw, Either Arm, or Epigastric Region. Source: J. Heuser / Wikimedia Commons / CC-BY-SA-3.0 / GNU Free Documentation License. Image at en.wikipedia.org/wiki/File:AMI_pain_front.png

Figure 2.6 Normal Sinus Rhythm: 60–100 Beats per Minute. Source: Glenlarson / Wikimedia Commons / Public Domain. Image at commons.wikimedia.org/wiki/File:12_lead_generated_sinus_rhythm.JPG

Figure 2.7 Sinus Tachycardia. Source: User:MoodyGroove / Wikimedia Commons / CC-BY-SA-3.0 / GNU Free Documentation License. Image at en.wikipedia.org/wiki/File:SinusTach.jpg

Figure 2.8 Abnormal Pattern—Ventricular Tachycardia. Source: Glenlarson, File:Lead II rhythm ventricular tachycardia Vtach VT.JPG. Public Domain. Image at commons.wikimedia.org/wiki/File:Lead_II_rhythm_ventricular_tachycardia_Vtach_VT.JPG

Figure 2.9 Sinus Bradycardia. Source: Glenlarson, File:12 lead sinus bradycardia.JPG. Public Domain. Image at commons.wikimedia.org/wiki/File:12_lead_sinus_bradycardia.JPG

Figure 2.10 Atrial Flutter. Source: James Heilman, MD / Wikimedia Commons / CC-BY-SA-3.0 / GNU Free Documentation License. Image at commons.wikimedia.org/wiki/File:_Atrial_flutter34.JPG

Figure 2.11 Ventricular Fibrillation. Source: Jer5150, File:Ventricular fibrillation.png, CC-BY-SA-3.0 / GNU Free Documentation License. Image at commons.wikimedia.org/wiki/File:Lead_II_rhythm_generated_ventricular_fibrilation_VF.JPG

Figure 2.12 Anterior Wall MI. Source: Glenlarson, File:12 lead generated anterior MI.JPG. Public Domain. Image at commons.wikimedia.org/wiki/File:AnteriorLateralMI.jpg

Figure 2.13 Chest X-ray. Sources: Mikael Häggström, Chikumaya / Wikimedia Commons / CC-BY-SA-3.0 GNU Free Documentation License. Image at en.wikipedia.org/wiki/File:_Chest_labeled.png

Figure 2.14 Chest X-ray with Enlarged Heart, and Fluid Accumulation. Source: James Heilman, MD / Wikimedia Commons / CC-BY-SA-3.0 / GNU Free Documentation License. Image at en.wikipedia.org/wiki/File:_Pulmonaryedema09.JPG

Pulmonary Edema
ByStefanie Kosman

Introduction

- Pulmonary edema is a condition in which a patient has difficulty breathing due to excess fluid in the lung(s). This fluid collects in the air sacs (alveoli) inside the lungs. (See Figures 2.15 and 2.16.)

- The three types of pulmonary edema include acute, chronic, and high-altitude.

  - **Acute**

    - ▶ Develops suddenly and has the most visible symptoms

    - ▶ This is a medical emergency because it can cause respiratory failure and the cardiovascular system to collapse.

  - **Chronic**

    - ▶ Develops over time

    - ▶ Not as deadly as the other two types, but it should still be taken seriously

  - **High-altitude**

    - ▶ Can occur in healthy individuals and is life-threatening

    - ▶ The two primary causes are ascending to a high altitude quickly and descending from a high altitude quickly.

    - ▶ Other factors: exposure to the cold, strenuous exercise, or previously having high altitude pulmonary edema (HAPE).

I. Anatomical Points

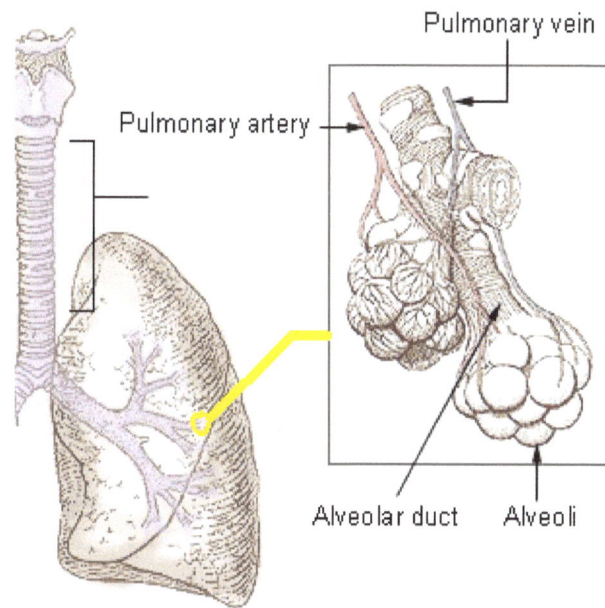

Figure 2.15 Left Lung Showing Gas Exchange. The enlarged section shows oxygen-depleted blood going to the lungs through the pulmonary arteries, picking up oxygen from the alveoli, and returning to the heart through the pulmonary veins.

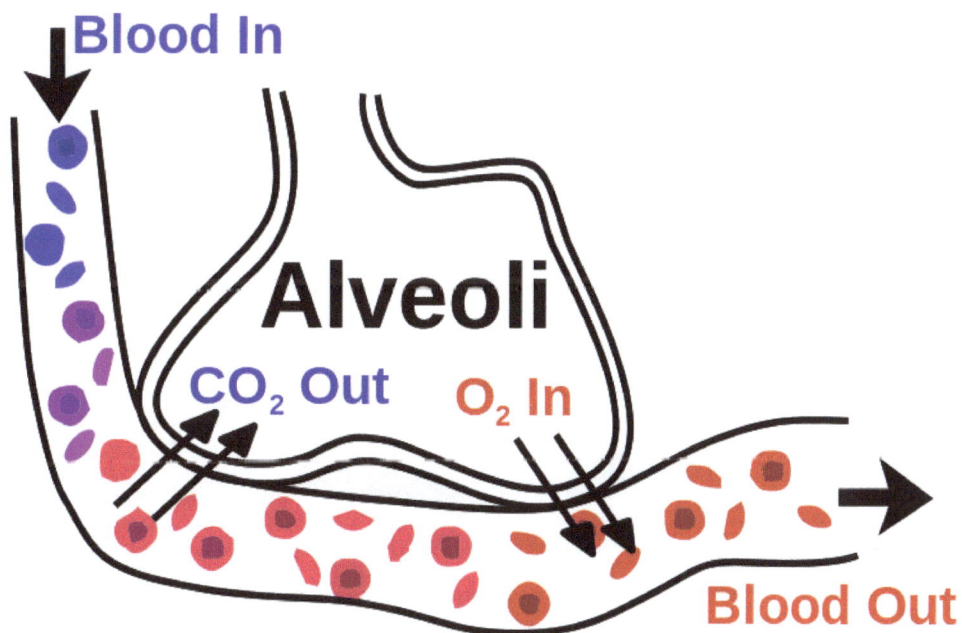

Figure 2.16 The Alveoli of the Lungs Exchanging Oxygen-Depleted Blood for Oxygen-Rich Blood.

II. Basic Physiology

- The causes of pulmonary edema can be separated into two main categories: cardiogenic (cardiac-related) and non-cardiogenic (pulmonary).

  ○ **Cardiogenic**

    ▶ Also known as congestive heart failure, and the most common cause of pulmonary edema

    ▶ Congestive heart failure occurs when the left ventricle is unable to pump enough blood from the lungs, increasing pressure in the left atrium.

    ▶ This also causes pressure to increase in the veins and capillaries of the lungs.

    ▶ The increased pressure of the capillaries forces some of the fluid out of the capillary walls into the alveoli.

    ▶ Common cardiogenic causes:

      ▷ Coronary artery disease: the narrowing or blocking of coronary arteries and small blood vessels

        ◆ This narrowing restricts blood flow to the heart, which can cause the heart to be deprived of nutrients and oxygen, thereby leading to a decreased ability to pump blood.

      ▷ Cardiomyopathy: diseases in which the heart muscle weakens

      ▷ Defective heart valve(s): heart valve(s) that fail to either close or open properly

      ▷ Hypertension (high blood pressure): the heart muscle thickens to compensate for the high blood pressure, eventually causing the heart muscle to weaken

  ○ **Pulmonary**

    ▶ The capillaries become more permeable, causing fluid to leak into the alveoli.

    ▶ Common pulmonary causes:

      ▷ Lung infections (e.g., pneumonia): edema occurs only in the swollen area

      ▷ Near-drowning

      ▷ Exposure to inhaled toxins, including chlorine or ammonia, or inhaling one's own vomit

      ▷ Smoke inhalation: the smoke damages the membrane that separates the air sacs and capillaries. This allows fluid to go into the air sacs.

      ▷ Kidney disease: excess fluid accumulates in the lungs due to the kidney's inability to remove waste

      ▷ Many adverse drug reactions, including to aspirin, chemotherapy drugs, heroin, or cocaine

▷ Acute respiratory distress syndrome (ARDS): a serious disorder that occurs when the lungs quickly fill with white blood cells and fluid.

◆ Many conditions can cause ARDS, including trauma, infections of the blood, pneumonia, and shock.

▷ Exercising at high-altitudes:

◆ Individuals who exercise without becoming acclimated to the new altitude are particularly at risk of developing HAPE, but individuals who have acclimated can also develop HAPE.

◆ Without proper treatment, this can be fatal.

III. Clinical Signs and Symptoms

- If the patient has any of the following signs, the condition is very serious:
  ○ A feeling of suffocating or having trouble breathing
  ○ A bluish or gray tone to the skin
  ○ Sweating combined with difficulty breathing
  ○ A severe drop in blood pressure that results in dizziness, weakness, and sweating
  ○ A wheezy, bubbly, or gasping sound when breathing
  ○ A sudden worsening of symptoms associated with pulmonary edema
- Symptoms may vary depending on the type.
  ○ **Acute pulmonary edema**
    ▶ Difficulty breathing that may increase when the patient lies down
    ▶ A feeling of suffocating or drowning
    ▶ Wheezing or gasping for air, an extreme shortness of breath
    ▶ Coughing up blood or frothy substance
    ▶ Anxiety or restlessness
    ▶ Pale skin
    ▶ Excessive sweating
    ▶ Chest pain (if caused by heart disease)
    ▶ A fast and irregular heartbeat
  ○ **Chronic pulmonary edema**
    ▶ Wheezing
    ▶ Fatigue

- ▶ More difficulty breathing when exercising or lying flat
- ▶ Awakening at night from shortness of breath. This goes away when sitting.
- ▶ Rapid weight gain (if the pulmonary edema is due to heart issues)
- ▶ Swelling of the legs and ankles
- ▶ Loss of appetite
- ○ **High-altitude pulmonary edema (HAPE)**
  - ▶ Shortness of breath and fatigue
  - ▶ Insomnia
  - ▶ Fluid retention
  - ▶ Headache and cough
  - ▶ Severe cases:
    - ▷ Wheezy respiration
    - ▷ Nauseated when resting
    - ▷ Productive cough, producing a frothy mucus
    - ▷ Purple or blue colored skin
    - ▷ Fog brained or cloudy consciousness

IV. Diagnostic Work-up

- ● Past medical history
  - ○ Shortness of breath during exertion
  - ○ Chest pain
  - ○ Waking from sleep due to respiratory distress
- ● Physical examination
  - ○ Listening to the lungs:
    - ▶ May hear sounds consistent with fluid accumulation
  - ○ X-ray reveals:
    - ▶ Opacities (areas impermeable to light, caused by fluid), which appear white on X-ray (Figure 2.17)
  - ○ Ultrasound shows:
    - ▶ Valve abnormalities
    - ▶ Pumping efficiency

▶ Heart muscle thickness

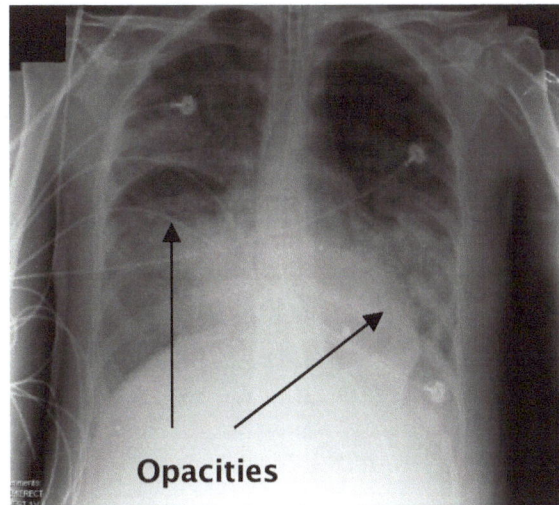

Figure 2.17 X-ray Showing Opacities (Areas of the Lungs Through Which Light Was Unable to Pass). This can occur when fluid accumulates in the lungs.

V. Treatment

- The treatment of the symptoms is similar for each type of pulmonary edema, but the treatment of the underlying cause varies.

- The primary treatment for pulmonary edema symptoms is the administration of oxygen, along with the following, in this order:

  ○ **For acute and chronic pulmonary edema**:

    ▶ The patient should be placed in an upright position and oxygen should be given through a face mask or nasal cannula (thin flexible tube) or by the use of a machine.

    ▶ Medications:

      ▷ Furosemide to reduce swelling and fluid retention:

        ◆ For patients who are not already on the medication, an initial dose of 20–40 mg should be given orally. Then 0.5–1.0 mg/kg of body weight intravenously.

        ◆ For patients already on the medication: 0.5–1.0 mg/kg of body weight intravenously

      ▷ Nitroglycerine to reduce the heart's workload: 0.4 mg under the tongue every 5 minutes

       ▷ Morphine to reduce anxiety and the feeling of shortness of breath, and to control pain: 1–4 mg intravenously until the respiratory status improves or the patient develops side effects (hypotension, altered mental status, or respiratory depression).

    ▶ Underlying cause should be diagnosed and treated.

       ▷ For example, antibiotics to treat infection or medication to control blood pressure

○ **For high-altitude pulmonary edema (HAPE):**

    ▶ The primary method is for the patient to descend the mountain immediately. This usually cures both HAPE and acute mountain sickness.

    ▶ If the patient is unable to descend, oxygen should be given.

    ▶ Nifedipine: the initial dose is 10 mg under the tongue, and then a 30-mg slow release tablet should be given.

VI. Complications

● If left untreated, pulmonary edema can cause harmful complications, or even death. Complications include:

  ○ Increased pressure in the pulmonary artery

  ○ Right ventricle failure

  ○ Pleural effusion (accumulation of fluid in the membranes that surround the lungs)

  ○ Swelling of the abdomen and legs

  ○ Congestion and swelling of the liver

VII. Prevention

● The main method is preventing cardiovascular disease. These steps can help reduce the risk:

  ○ Control blood pressure:

    ▶ The resting blood pressure should be between 120/80 mm Hg and 140/90 mm Hg.

    ▶ Most people can lower their blood pressure by maintaining an ideal weight, exercising regularly, and limiting sodium intake.

  ○ Manage blood cholesterol:

    ▶ High cholesterol may cause plaque (fatty deposits) to form in the arteries, restricting blood flow through the arteries. This increases blood pressure and the risk of vascular disease.

    ▶ Lifestyle changes can help lower cholesterol.

  ○ Do not smoke.

References

Altitude Diseases. Merck Manuals.
www.merckmanuals.com/professional/injuries_poisoning/altitude_sickness/altitude_sickness.html?qt=pulmonary%20edema&alt=sh#v1115101

Arnold, J. Malcolm O. Pulmonary Edema. Merck Manuals.
www.merckmanuals.com/professional/cardiovascular_disorders/heart_failure/pulmonary_edema.html

Borden Institute: Office of the Surgeon General.
www.bordeninstitute.army.mil/published_volumes/harshEnv2/HE2ch25.pdf

Johnson, Maryl R. Acute Pulmonary Edema. *Current Treatment Options in Cardiovascular Medicine* 1, no. 3 (1999): 269–277.

Pulmonary Edema. Mayo Clinic. www.mayoclinic.com/health/pulmonary-edema/DS00412

Pulmonary Edema. Medline Plus. www.nlm.nih.gov/medlineplus/ency/article/000140.htm

Figure 2.15 Left Lung Showing Gas Exchange Source: National Cancer Institute / Wikimedia Commons / Public Domain. Image at commons.wikimedia.org/wiki/File:Illu_bronchi_lungs.jpg

Figure 2.16 The Alveoli of the Lungs Exchanging Oxygen-Depleted Blood for Oxygen-Rich Blood. Source: helix84 / Wikimedia Commons / CC-BY-SA-3.0 / GNU Free Documentation License. Image at commons.wikimedia.org/w/index.php?title=File:Alveoli.svg&page=1

Figure 2.17 X-ray Showing Opacities (Areas of the Lungs Through Which Light Was Unable to Pass). Source: Samir, Delldot / Wikimedia Commons / CC-BY-SA-3.0 / GNU Free Documentation License. Image at commons.wikimedia.org/wiki/File:AARDS_X-ray_cropped.jpg

Congestive Heart Failure

By Robert R. Simon, MD

Introduction

- Congestive heart failure (left side heart failure) occurs when the heart cannot effectively pump oxygenated blood to the rest of the body.

- There are four stages of heart failure, ranging from 1 (mild, no limitations on activity) to 4 (severe, unable to engage in physical activity without discomfort; symptoms occur even when the patient is resting; patient may need a transplant).

- The following disorders can cause end-stage (stage 4) heart failure:

  - Consistent high blood pressure (malignant hypertension)

  - A heart attack (myocardial infarction)

  - Inflammation of the heart muscle (myocarditis)

  - The heart muscle becomes weak, enlarged, or too thick (dilated and hypertrophic cardiomyopathies)

  - Severe anemia, vitamin B1/thiamine deficiency, and hyperthyroidism

I. Anatomy and Basic Physiology

- Congestive heart failure (CHF) can occur because the heart is too weak or enlarged, or the heart muscle is too thick.

- Congestive heart failure can lead to a buildup of fluid or swelling in the lungs (pulmonary edema), the peritoneal cavity (ascites) and the legs and feet (peripheral edema).

- The two types of congestive heart failure that require immediate hospitalization are chronic heart failure and acute decompensated heart failure (a rapid worsening of the symptoms of heart failure).

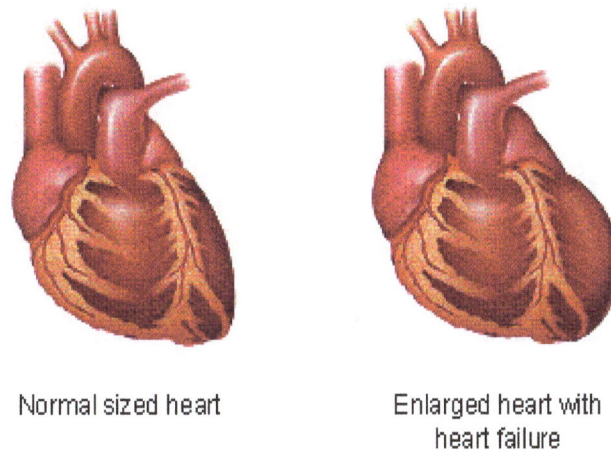

Normal sized heart   Enlarged heart with
                          heart failure

Figure 2.18 Normal Heart vs. an Enlarged Heart.

II. Clinical Signs and Symptoms

- Common signs and symptoms of congestive heart failure (left-sided heart failure) may include:

  ○ Shortness of breath during activity and sleep*

  ○ Bright or dark red streaks of blood in mucus from the lungs, nose, or mouth*

  ○ Enlarged heart*

  ○ Cool and pale blue fingers, lips, or extremities*

  ○ Complaints of not "getting enough air" or being "out of breath" during an activity or when sleeping

  ○ Suddenly awake from sleep, breathless with coughing and wheezing (whistling sound)

  ○ Frequent desire to sleep sitting up

  ○ Crackling/clicking heard at the base of one or both lungs when listening with stethoscope

  ○ A third heart sound (S3 gallop) after the normal "lub-dub" (S1-S2) heart sounds

  ○ Decreased urine output—less than 500 mL of urine in 24 hours

  ○ Fatigue

*Note that the first four signs and symptoms occur in patients with severe pulmonary edema.

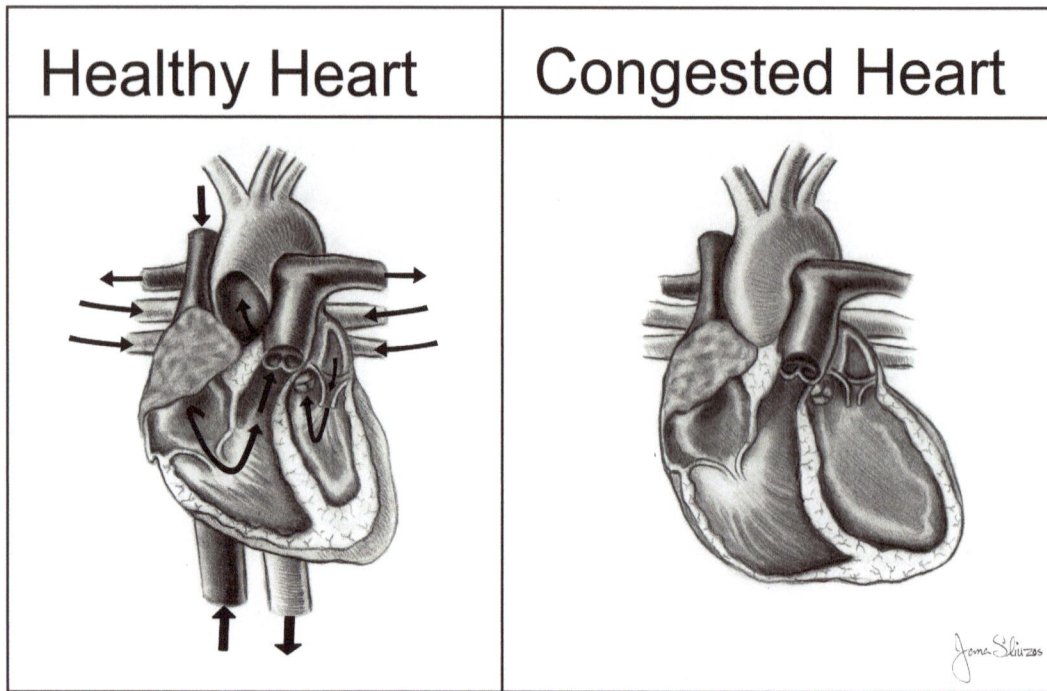

Figure 2.19 Healthy Heart Compared to Congested Heart.

- Pulmonary edema often develops before right ventricular (heart) failure.
  - Left side heart failure can lead to right side heart failure.
- The signs and symptoms of right side heart failure include the following:
  - Fatigue
  - Enlarged liver and spleen
  - Accumulation of fluid in the peritoneal cavity (ascites). The patient will have a swollen abdomen.
  - Distended jugular or neck veins

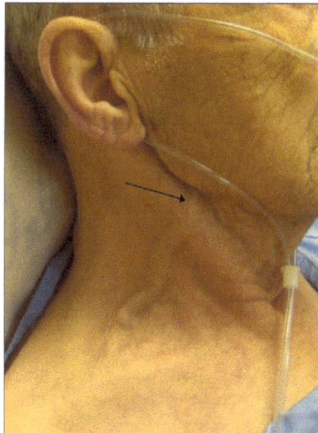

Figure 2.20 Distended Jugular Vein.

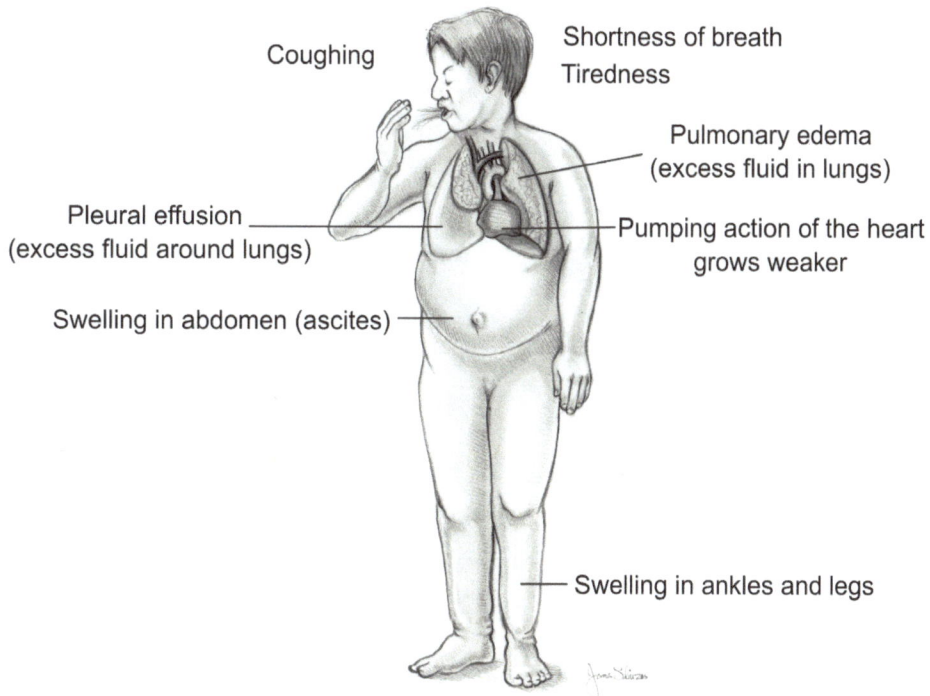

Coughing

Shortness of breath
Tiredness

Pulmonary edema
(excess fluid in lungs)

Pleural effusion
(excess fluid around lungs)

Pumping action of the heart
grows weaker

Swelling in abdomen (ascites)

Swelling in ankles and legs

Figure 2.21 Common Signs and Symptoms of Congestive Heart Failure.

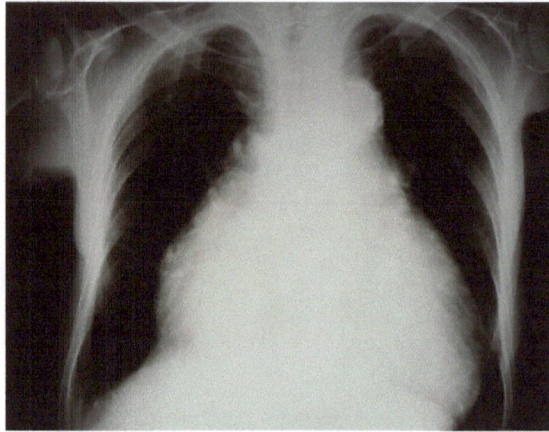

Figure 2.22 Chest X-ray of Cardiomegaly.

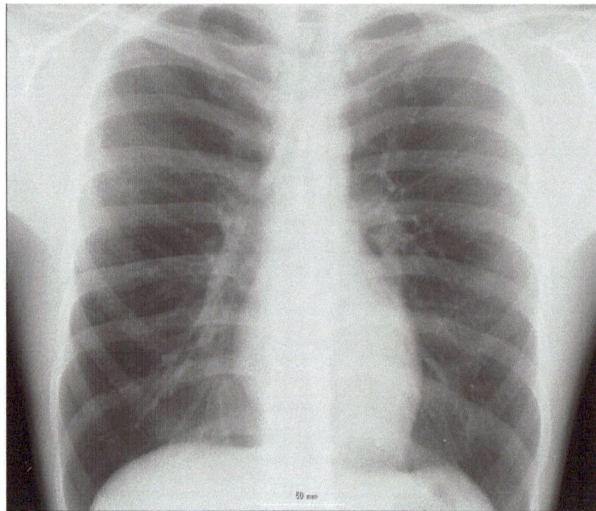

Figure 2.23 Chest X-ray of Normal-Sized Heart.

III. Diagnostic Work-up

● Complete a chest X-ray and blood tests to confirm the presence of heart failure and rule out primary pulmonary disease or other blood disorders like sepsis (blood infection).

● Look for these signs:

○ Enlarged heart

○ Vascular redistribution: blood flow to the upper lungs increases (lungs appear larger)

○ The heart's width is larger than half the width of the rib cage (thoracic diameter).

You can encounter a normal sized heart in acute myocardial infarction.

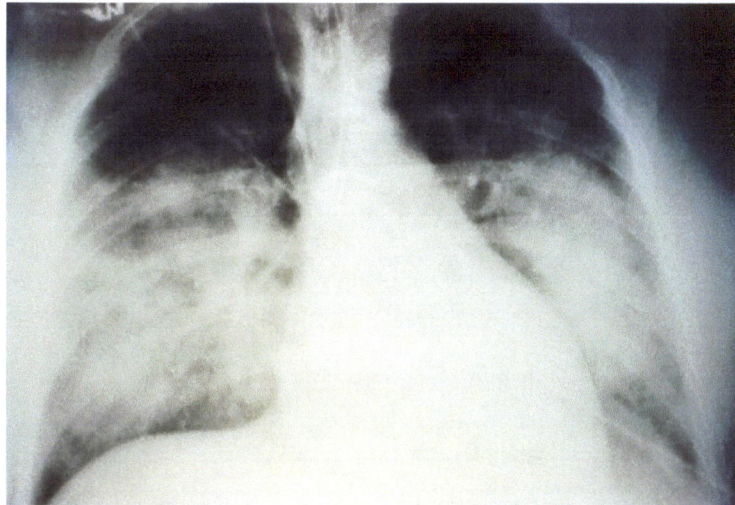

Figure 2.24 Chest X-ray Showing Pulmonary Edema.

● Blood tests

○ Complete blood count, to help rule out coexisting or alternate conditions like anemia (low red blood cells) and sepsis

○ Low blood sodium level indicates severe heart failure, but you should look for excessive sweating, as this can also be a cause of low sodium

○ Serum electrolytes, blood urea nitrogen (BUN) and creatinine to evaluate kidney function and to determine which therapy (diuretics and/or angiotensin converting enzyme [ACE] inhibitors) to initiate for treatment

▶ Problem if BUN reaches 100 mg/dL and the serum creatinine reaches 8 mg/dL

○ A liver function test in case the liver is enlarged (hepatic congestion)

Table 2.8 Blood Electrolyte Levels

Electrolyte	Normal Results Range	Abnormal Range	Possible Interventions
Potassium (K⁺)	3.6 to 5.4 mEq/L	<2.8 mEq/L or >6 mEq/L Signs of low potassium: muscle aches, weakness, palpitations. Signs of high potassium: tall, peaked T waves on ECG, widened QT interval, palpitations.	Patients with low potassium may need only oral potassium replacement (20–40 mEq by mouth 2–4 times a day); however, if K⁺ <2.5 mEq/L, start with 40 mEq IV over 4 hours with continuous cardiac monitoring and follow-up testing of serum potassium levels.
Magnesium (Mg⁺⁺)	>1.7 mEq/L	<1.6 mEq/L Signs of low magnesium: muscular weakness and tremors progressing to paresthesias (sensations of burning, numbing, tingling, or prickling), tetany (a condition usually related to low calcium, characterized by cramps/spasms of hands and feet), and seizures. Premature ventricular contractions (PVCs), prolonged QT interval and prominent U waves after T waves on continuous ECG.	If 1.5 to 2 mEq/L, give 2 g magnesium sulfate IV over 1 hour If 0.9 to 1.4 mEq/L, give 2 g magnesium sulfate IV over 1 hour for 2 doses *Note: often, low potassium and low calcium will not resolve until low magnesium is addressed.*
Sodium (Na⁺)	136 to 143 mEq/L	<120 mEq/L or >160 mEq/L	Fluid restriction to 2 L/day can "raise" sodium levels through hemoconcentration. Fluid status maintenance of congestive heart failure generally requires restriction of dietary sodium to 2–3 g/daily (which reduces fluid retention).

Electrolyte	Normal Results Range	Abnormal Range	Possible Interventions
Calcium (Ca++)	8.5 to 10.5 mg/dL	<6 mg/dL and >12.9 mg/dL	For low calcium, give calcium chloride: 1 g IV over 10 minutes, preferably in a central line or calcium gluconate: 3 g IV over 10 minutes
Chloride Cl-	98 to 108 mmol/L	Trends in the same direction as sodium and is corrected when sodium is corrected.	
Carbon dioxide (CO_2)	22 to 31 mmol/L	Measures the amount of bicarbonate in the blood.	

Table 2.9 Tests for Kidney and Liver Function

Kidney and Liver Function Tests	
Creatinine Levels to Assess Kidney Damage	
Creatinine level	*Kidney's approximate loss of nephrons (functional units of the kidney)*
0.6 to 1.5 mg	up to 50% loss possible
1.6 to 4.6 mg	>50% loss possible
4.7 to 9.9 mg	up to 75% loss possible
>10 mg	90% loss possible, *end-stage kidney disease*
Liver Function Tests	
LFT (liver function test)	*Normal range*
Albumin (serum)	3.4 to 5 grams/dL (marker of nutrition status)
Total serum bilirubin	0.1 to 1.3 mg/dL (adults)
Direct (conjugated) bilirubin [Adult only]	0.0 to 0.3mg/dL (bile ducts in liver may be blocked)

Kidney and Liver Function Tests	
Liver Function Tests	
LFT (liver function test)	*Normal range*
Indirect (unconjugated) bilirubin [Adult only]	0.2 to 0.8 mg/dL: total bilirubin minus direct bilirubin (increase may indicate liver cell dysfunction)
AST (Aspartate aminotransferase) [Adult only]	5 to 38 IU/L (increase may indicate liver damage)
ALT (Alanine aminotransferase) [Adult only]	7 to 50 IU/L (increase may indicate liver damage)
ALP (Alkaline phosphatase) [Adult only]	30 to 130 ImU/mL (increase may indicate biliary tract problem)
GGT (Gamma-glutamyltransferase)	Men = 15 to 70 U/L; Women = 5 to 45 U/L (increase may indicate heavy alcohol use)
Total serum protein [Adult only]	6 to 8.2 grams/dL

###

IV. Treatment

Table 2.10 Treatment for Congestive Heart Failure

Drug Name (Generic/Trade)	Dosage	Comments
Nitroglycerin (vasodilator/ widening blood vessels therapy)	*Ointment*: 1/2 to 2 inches applied every 4–6 hours, squeezed as thin layer onto paper, and spread onto non-hairy area of skin *Capsule*: 2.5–9 mg administered 2–3 times per day 1–2 hours after a meal	Used to increase the blood supply to the heart. Not for patients with low blood pressure.

Drug Name (Generic/Trade)	Dosage	Comments
Dopamine (for patients with low blood pressure [BP], increases force of contractions)	*Medium dose:* 5–15 mcg/kg/minute IV may increase blood flow to kidneys, cardiac output, heart rate, and cardiac contractility *High dose:* 20–50 mcg/kg/minute IV may increase BP and stimulate vasoconstriction (narrowing of blood vessels) Titrate to response	Used in severe heart failure; reserved for patients with moderate hypotension (systolic BP 70–90 mm Hg). Typically, moderate or higher doses are used
Supplemental oxygen	2–6 L/minute by nasal cannula, increasing to 10–15 L/minute by non-rebreather mask as needed.	As needed to increase oxygenation of the heart muscle

Diuretics (to reduce blood volume and pulmonary edema)	Fluid restriction (oral and/or IV). Keep strict intake and output record.
	
	Diuretic, potassium non-sparing (do not use if patient is hypotensive [has low blood pressure], oliguric [low urine volume], or anuric [absence of urine]):
	
	• **Furosemide**
	  ¤ Oral: initial 20–80 mg/day, may repeat in 6–8 hours.
	    ◊ Maximum of 600 mg/day
	  ¤ IM/IV push: 20–40 mg slowly over 1–2 minutes
	    ◊ May repeat in 1–2 hours; or
	    ◊ Increase dose by 20 mg until desired response
	    ◊ This individualized dose may be given 1–2 times/day
	  ¤ IVPB: dose in 50mL normal saline, maximum rate 4 mg/minute
	• **Bumetanide** (only use if patient is not allergic to sulfonamides)
	  ¤ Oral: 0.5–2 mg dose (1–2 times/day)
	    ◊ Maximum dose 10 mg/day
	  ¤ IM/IV push: 0.5–1 mg dose given slowly
	    ◊ May repeat in 2–3 hours for up to 2 doses if needed.
	    ◊ Maximum dose 10 mg/day
	  ¤ Continuous IV: 0.1–1 mg/hour
		1st-line diuretic therapy: loop diuretic (furosemide, bumetanide, torsemide) in lowest dose that is effective, either once or twice a day.
		
		Can be used up to 3–4 times a day if necessary
		
		Oral form provides better response on an empty stomach.

Drug Name (Generic/Trade)	Dosage	Comments
Decrease sodium and fluid intake	Limit sodium intake to a maximum 2 g daily	As needed to reduce fluid buildup in the body
ACE inhibitors (decrease heart workload and help restore blood to extremities)	**Captopril** *Initial dose*: 6.25–12.5 mg by mouth every 8 hours, along with cardiac glycoside (digoxin) and diuretic therapy *Target therapy*: 50 mg every 8 hours 450 mg/day maximum	Take on empty stomach, 1–2 hours after meals DO NOT USE ACE inhibitors with spironolactone (a diuretic)
Digoxin (increases strength of contractions)	**Loading-dose regimen** (large dose in beginning of a series) *IV*: 0.4–0.6 mg once, then may cautiously give additional doses of 0.1–0.3 mg every 6–8 hours until adequate effect; not to exceed 0.008–0.015 mg/kg total. *By mouth*: 0.5–0.75 mg once, then cautiously give additional doses of 0.125–0.375 mg every 6–8 hours until adequate effect is achieved, up to 0.75–1.25 mg (for 70-kg patient) *Maintenance*: 0.125–0.5 mg/day IV or by mouth	
Morphine sulfate (reduces pulmonary edema and pain)	**Oral** *Immediate release*: 5–30 mg every 4 hours *Oral solution*: 10–20 mg every 4 hours *Sustained release*: 15–30 mg SR every 8–12 hours	

###

V. Complications

- Acute decompensated heart failure
- Cardiogenic shock (condition in which the heart can't pump as much blood as the body needs)
- Renal failure (kidney failure)
- Electrolyte disturbances
- Respiratory failure

- Adverse reactions: some medications can interact with each other and make heart failure worse

  ○ **DO NOT USE** ACE inhibitors with spironolactone (a diuretic).

  ○ **DO NOT USE** aspirin with ACE inhibitors, diuretics or beta blockers.

  ○ Patients on warfarin, digoxin, and beta blockers should have routine blood work-up.

  ○ Diabetics with CHF should not take the oral anti-diabetic drug metformin, due to potential complications involving lactic acidosis.

  ○ Antihistamines, which have potential to induce cardiac arrhythmias, and sodium bicarbonate products like Fleet PhosPho soda, which contain high sodium, can exacerbate CHF

  ○ Advise patients to stop drinking caffeinated drinks like tea and coffee.

VI. Prevention

- High risk of heart failure is associated with disease states like high blood pressure, diabetes, heart disease (coronary artery disease), and obesity. To manage risk, patients should:

  ○ Eat a healthy diet of fruits, vegetables, and whole grains like multigrain bread and oatmeal, and avoid fatty foods with excess sodium (salt).

  ○ Stop smoking, and stop excessive alcohol consumption; moderate alcohol consumption is 5 drinks/week.

  ○ Make a plan with their cardiologist for an appropriate schedule of regular exercise, such as 30–60 minutes of daily walking.

  ○ Get vaccinated: pneumococcal pneumonia vaccine, influenza vaccine

Special thanks to contributor Madhu Prasad.

References

Bacterial Pneumonia. eMedicineHealth.
www.emedicinehealth.com/bacterial_pneumonia/article_em.htm

Conditions in Depth: Hypertension. BeliefNet.
www.beliefnet.com/healthandhealing/getcontent.aspx?cid=19591

Congestive Heart Failure. Humanity First: Serving Mankind.
medicinembbs.blogspot.com/2010/12/congestive-heart-failure.html

Congestive Heart Failure. MedicaLook.
www.medicalook.com/Heart_diseases/Congestive_heart_failure.html

Congestive Heart Failure. Pharmacy and Drugs.
www.pharmacy-and-drugs.com/Heart_diseases/Congestive_heart_failure.html

Heart Failure Treatment and Management. Medscape.
emedicine.medscape.com/article/163062-treatment#aw2aab6b6b2

Pneumonia. Mayo Clinic. www.mayoclinic.com/health/pneumonia/DS00135

Pneumonia. PubMedHealth. www.ncbi.nlm.nih.gov/pubmedhealth/PMH0001200/

Pneumonia in Chidren. Boston Children's Hospital.
www.childrenshospital.org/az/Site1457/mainpageS1457P0.html

Potassium Chloride. Medscape. reference.medscape.com/drug/kdur-slow-k-potassium-chloride-344450

Routine Blood and Urine Testing. CHF Patients. www.chfpatients.com/tests/routine_tests.htm

What Is Pneumonia? eHealthMD. ehealthmd.com/library/pneumonia/pnm_whatis.html

Figure 2.18 Normal Heart vs. an Enlarged Heart. Source: US Food and Drug Administration / Public Domain. Image at
www.fda.gov/ohrms/dockets/ac/05/briefing/2005-4149b1_01_DRAFT%20PATIENT%20INFO%20BOOKLET_files/image002.gif

Figure 2.19 Healthy Heart Compared to Congested Heart. Source: Jana Sliuzas, Medical illustrator.

Figure 2.20 Distended Jugular Vein. Source: James Heilman, MD / Wikimedia Commons / CC-BY-SA-3.0. Image at commons.wikimedia.org/wiki/File:Elevated_JVP.JPG

Figure 2.21 Common Signs and Symptoms of Congestive Heart Failure. Source: Jana Sliuzas, Medical illustrator.

Figure 2.22 Chest X-Ray of Cardiomegaly. Source: Nevit Dilmen / Wikimedia Commons / CC-BY-SA-3.0 / GNU Free Documentation License. Image at commons.wikimedia.org/wiki/File:Rad_1300124.JPG

Figure 2.23 Chest X-ray of Normal Sized Heart. Source: Chikumaya / Wikimedia Commons / CC-BY-SA-3.0 / GNU Free Documentation License. Image at commons.wikimedia.org/wiki/File:Chest.png

Figure 2.24 Chest X-ray Showing Pulmonary Edema. Source: CDC / D. Loren Ketai, MD / Wikimedia Commons / Public Domain. Image at commons.wikimedia.org/wiki/File:6077_lores.jpg

Chapter 3:

Arrhythmias

Sinus Node Dysfunction (SND) and Atrioventricular (AV) Block

By Marian M. Houtman

Introduction

- The **sinoatrial node** (SA node) is also called the "pacemaker" of the heart.
  - The SA node is a collection of cardiac muscle fibers in which muscle contractions are initiated.
  - The SA node determines the heart rate, the number of times the heart beats per minute.
- The **atrioventricular node** (AV node) relays impulses from the SA node to the ventricles, causing contraction and ejection of blood into the pulmonary artery.
- The pattern of the heart rhythm is usually regular, but may be irregular (called an arrhythmia) if some impulses are delayed.

I. Anatomical Points

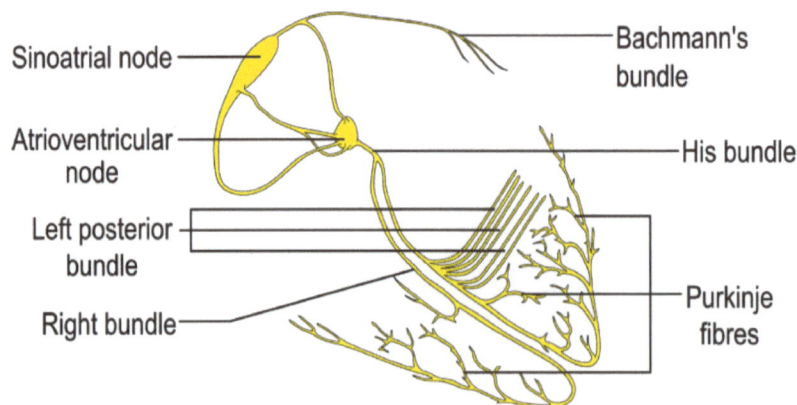

Figure 3.1 Electrical Conduction System of the Heart.

II. Basic Physiology

- The electrical conduction system controls the rate and rhythm of the heartbeat.
- Some people are born with an abnormal rhythm of the heart (congenital), whereas others may develop heart block (a type of arrhythmia) during their lifetime (acquired).

- Acquired heart block is caused by damage to the heart muscle or conduction system due to surgery, disease, medication, or other causes.

- Congenital heart block is less common than acquired heart block.

- An electrocardiogram (EKG/ECG) test is used to diagnose a heart block.

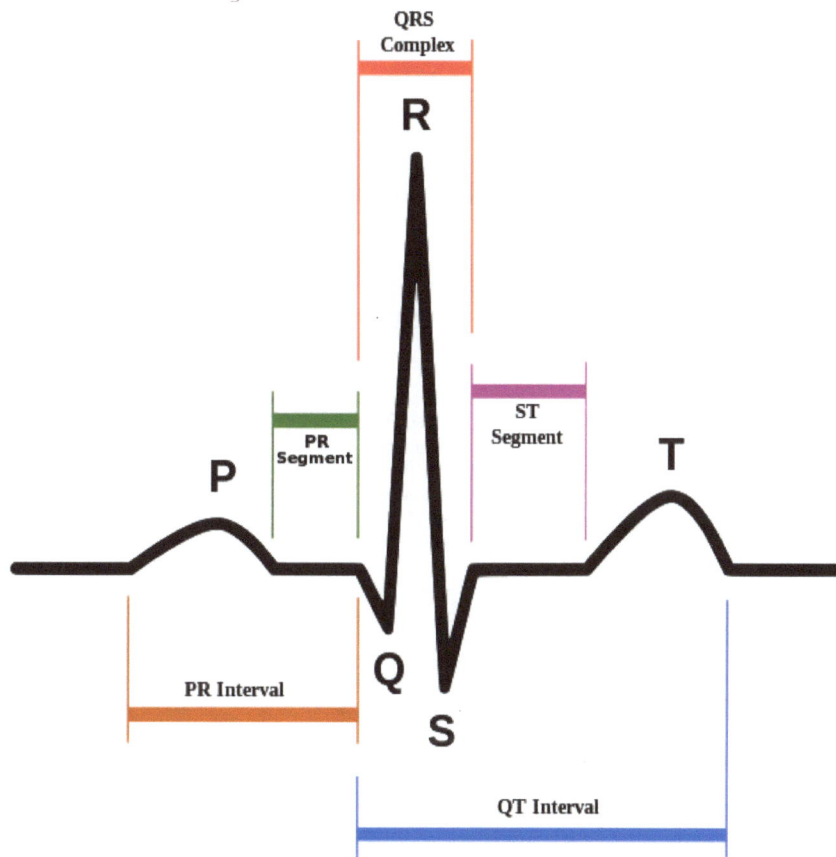

Figure 3.2 Normal Impulse Conduction.

- Normal impulse conduction
  - **P wave:** electrical depolarization of atria
  - **PR interval:** atrial contraction
  - **QRS complex:** electrical depolarization of ventricles
  - **ST segment:** ventricles contract
  - **T wave:** repolarization of ventricles

III. Clinical Signs and Symptoms

- Sinus node dysfunction is also called sick sinus syndrome.

- Sinus node dysfunction is a conduction defect in which the electrical impulse is slowed or disrupted as it moves from the atria (upper chamber) to the ventricle (lower chamber) of the heart.

- Disorder types:
  - 1st degree
  - 2nd degree type I
  - 2nd degree type II
  - 3rd degree

- **1st-degree heart block**: delay of signal stimulating ventricles to contract
  - Definition
    - ▶ Prolonged PR interval on EKG, >200 msec (0.20 seconds)
    - ▶ 1P wave: 1 QRS ratio
    - ▶ Delay in conduction from SA node through AV junction.
    - ▶ No missed beats
    - ▶ Every atria beat (upper chamber) is conducted to the ventricle (lower chamber)
    - ▶ Regular ventricular rate
  - Causes
    - ▶ Atrioventricular node disease
    - ▶ Vagal nerve stimulation; anti-adrenaline effect slows the heart
    - ▶ Acute MI, particularly acute inferior wall MI
    - ▶ Myocarditis: inflammation of the heart muscle, which can be secondary to the flu
    - ▶ Electrical disturbance (potassium level <3.5 mEQ/liter, magnesium level <1.7mg/dL)
    - ▶ Athletic training
    - ▶ Coronary artery disease (CAD): narrowing of the blood vessels to the heart
    - ▶ Idiopathic (unknown cause) degenerative disease of the conduction system
    - ▶ Drugs: some antiarrhythmics, digoxin, magnesium
    - ▶ Mitral aortic valve calcification
    - ▶ Infectious disease: endocarditis, tuberculosis, diphtheria, rheumatic fever, Lyme disease
    - ▶ Collagen vascular disease: arthritis, lupus, scleroderma
  - Symptoms
    - ▶ Usually no symptoms

- **2nd-degree heart block, type I AV block** (also called Mobitz I or Wenckebach AV block): disturbance or delay of impulse conduction to the ventricles through the AV node (Figure 3.3.)

  o Definition

    ▶ PR interval increases each beat until a QRS is dropped (P wave abruptly not followed by QRS complex)

    ▶ Wide QRS complex is frequently associated with a block to His bundle.

    ▶ A normal QRS complex width suggests that the block is above His bundle.

    ▶ A narrow QRS complex without underlying cardiac disease is usually a conductive disorder, rarely related to structural abnormality

    ▶ 1 P wave: 1 QRS complex ratio is not maintained

    ▶ P wave is not conducted through the His–Purkinje system

    ▶ There is progressive shortening of the R-R interval (the interval from the peak of one QRS complex to the peak of the next) prior to the missed beat

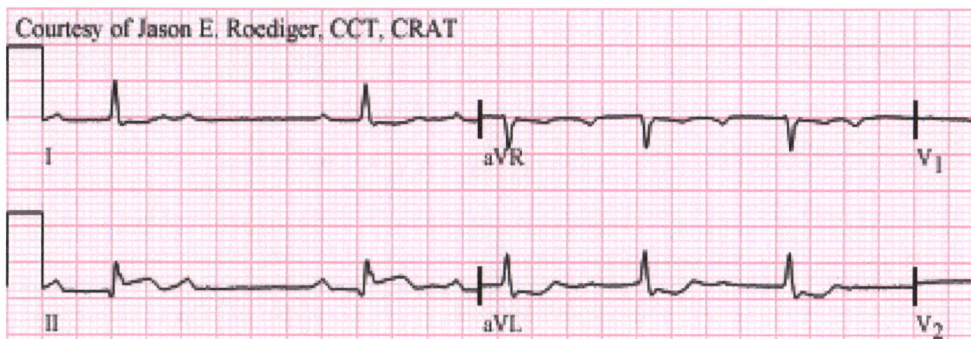

Figure 3.3 EKG Diagram of a 2nd-degree Type I Heart Block (Wenckebach).

- **2nd-degree heart block, type II AV block** (Mobitz II): disturbance or interruption of impulse conduction to the ventricles through the AV node (Figure 3.4)

  o Definition

    ▶ PR interval does not change

    ▶ Some QRS complexes are missing without warning

    ▶ All P waves are present, but QRS is missing every third or fourth beat

    ▶ PR interval may be normal (120–200 msec) or prolonged (>200 msec)

    ▶ The shortest PR interval is immediately following the missing QRS complex

    ▶ P-P intervals (the distance between consecutive P waves) are constant since atrial rhythm is regular

▶ May progress to a 3rd-degree heart block

○ Causes

▶ Conduction disturbances in AV node (70% cases)

▶ Abnormality below AV node in His bundle or both bundle branches (30% cases)

▶ Vagal increases caused by pain, carotid massage, hypersensitive carotid sinus, young patients, or athletes at rest

▶ Drugs: digoxin, beta blockers, calcium channel blockers, antiarrhythmics

▶ Inflammatory disease: endocarditis, myocarditis, Lyme disease, rheumatic fever

▶ Amyloidosis, sarcoidosis, hemochromatosis

▶ Malignancies, Hodgkin's lymphoma

▶ Metabolic and endocrine disorders: Addison's disease, hyperthyroidism

▶ Ankylosing spondylitis, rheumatoid arthritis

▶ Cardiac tumor

▶ Trauma

▶ Acute MI

▶ Complications following other surgical cardiac interventions

○ Symptoms: no symptoms or may have dizziness, fainting

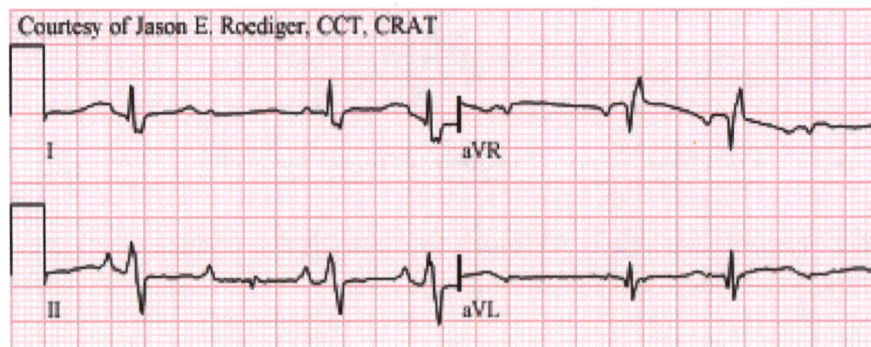

Figure 3.4 EKG Diagram of a 2nd-Degree, Type II Heart Block.

● **3rd-degree heart block**: complete block; no conduction through the AVN (Figure 3.5)

○ Definition

▶ No correlation between P waves and QRS complexes

▷ Means there is no communication between atria and ventricles.

▶ A narrow QRS complex at a rate of 30–40 beats per minute

○ Causes

- ▶ Lack of blood to cardiac muscle

- ▶ Acute myocardial infarction

- ▶ Congenital (at birth)

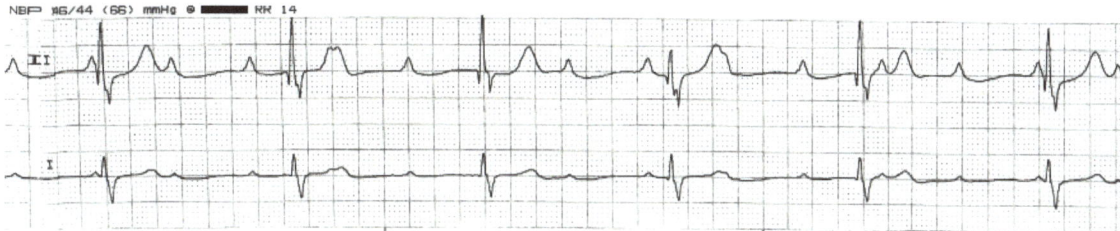

Figure 3.5 EKG Diagram of 3rd-Degree Heart Block.

IV. Treatment

- **1st-degree heart block**

  ○ Treat underlying cause for the 1st-degree heart block (avoid AV nodal blocking agents: beta-blockers, calcium channel blockers, digitalis)

  ○ Benign rhythm, does not require treatment

- **2nd-degree heart block type I AV block** (Mobitz I, Wenckebach)

  ○ No treatment, or determine underlying cause and treat

  ○ Changing drug, reducing or discontinuing dosage may restore normal rhythm.

- **2nd-degree heart block, type II AV block** (Mobitz II) or **3rd-degree heart block**

  ○ Must be treated

    - ▶ Without symptoms:

      ▷ Determine cause and treat

      ▷ Changing drug, reducing or discontinuing dosage may restore normal rhythm.

    - ▶ With bradycardia, hypotension, and other symptoms:

      ▷ Standard advanced cardiovascular life support (ACLS) guidelines

        ◆ Atropine 0.5 mg IV push every 3–5 minutes up to 3 mg

        ◆ Do not delay transcutaneous pacing

        ◆ Start dopamine infusion at 5 mcg/kg/minute and titrate to improved heart rate and blood pressure

      ▷ If chest pain, use appropriate anti-ischemic protocol.

▷ Assess medication dosages/levels.

▷ Consider placement of internal pacemaker at institution with cardiologist and interventional heart catheterization lab.

▷ Pacemaker: a battery-operated device about the size of a cell phone that is implanted under the collarbone.

◆ Wires from the device are threaded through veins and into the heart.

◆ Electrodes at the end of the wires are attached to heart tissues.

◆ The pacemaker monitors heart rate and generates electrical impulses as necessary to maintain an appropriate rate.

V. Complications

● Atrial fibrillation, atrial flutter, or other cardiac dysfunction

● Exercise intolerance

● Syncope (fainting)

● Falls

● Stroke

● Congestive heart failure

● Sudden cardiac death

References

Alaeddini, Jamshid. First-Degree Atrioventricular Block. Medscape. emedicine.medscape.com/article/161829-overview#aw2aab6b2b3

Sovari, Ali A. Second-Degree Atrioventricular Block Treatment and Management. Medscape. emedicine.medscape.com/article/161919-treatment

What Is Heart Block? NIH: National Heart, Lung, and Blood Institute. www.nhlbi.nih.gov/health/health-topics/topics/hb/

Yang, Yingbo. Sinus Node Dysfunction. Medscape. emedicine.medscape.com/article/158064-overview#aw2aab6b2b5aa

Figure 3.1 Electrical Conduction System of the Heart. Source: Madhero88 / Wikimedia Commons / CC-BY-SA-3.0. Image at commons.wikimedia.org/wiki/File:ConductionsystemoftheheartwithouttheHeart.png

Figure 3.2 Normal Impulse Conduction. Source: Anthony Atkielski / Wikimedia Commons / Public Domain. Image at upload.wikimedia.org/wikipedia/commons/5/53/SinusRhythmLabels.png

Figure 3.3 EKG Diagram of a 2nd-degree, Type I Heart Block (Wenckebach). Source: Jer5150 / Wikimedia Commons / CC-BY-SA-3.0. Image at en.wikipedia.org/wiki/ File:Type_I_A-V_block_5-to-4_Wenckebach_periods.png

Figure 3.4 EKG Diagram of a 2nd-Degree, Type II Heart Block. Source: Jer5150 / Wikimedia Commons / CC-BY-SA-3.0. Image at commons.wikimedia.org/wiki/File:Sinus_rhythm_with_3-to-2_and_2-to-1_Type_II_A-V_block.png

Figure 3.5 EKG Diagram of 3rd-Degree Heart Block. Source: MoodyGroove / Wikimedia Commons / Public Domain. Image at en.wikipedia.org/wiki/File:CHB.jpg

Bundle Branch Block

By Marian M. Houtman and Dawn Johnston

Introduction

- A bundle branch block (BBB) is a type of conduction block involving partial or complete interruption of the flow of electrical impulses through the right or left bundle branches of the heart (see Figure 3.6).

- This can make it harder for the heart to pump blood effectively.

Table 3.1 Common Causes and Risk Factors for BBB

Right Bundle Branch Block (RBBB)	Left Bundle Branch Block (LBBB)
Congenital factors (present from birth)	Anatomic malformations
Prior heart surgery	Abnormalities of the conduction system
Prenatal exposure to human immunodeficiency virus (HIV)	Prior heart surgery
Myocarditis	Thickening of left ventricular walls
Congestive heart failure	Left ventricular disease
Atrial septal defect	Conduction disease
Ebstein abnormality (congenital heart defect)	Myocarditis
Cardiomyopathy	Cardiomyopathy
Duchenne muscular dystrophy (a hereditary X-linked myopathy, or muscle disease)	Hemochromatosis (too much iron in the body)
Myotonic dystrophy, characterized by muscular dystrophy, myotonias, frontal balding, cataracts	Sclerodegenerative diseases
Kearns-Sayre syndrome (rare)	Myocardial infarction

Right Bundle Branch Block (RBBB)	Left Bundle Branch Block (LBBB)
Brugada syndrome—channelopathy mediated by the SCN5A gene	Aortic valve endocarditis
Pulmonary embolism (acute condition)	Rheumatic fever with aortic valve involvement
Arrhythmogenic right ventricular cardiomyopathy (RBBB is diagnostic characteristic)	Perinatal exposure to HIV type
Blunt chest trauma—RBBB is associated with past chest trauma	
Polymyositis (inflammation of several muscles, which includes myopathy)	Wolff–Parkinson–White syndrome
Note: Left anterior fascicular block may have RBBB as well	

###

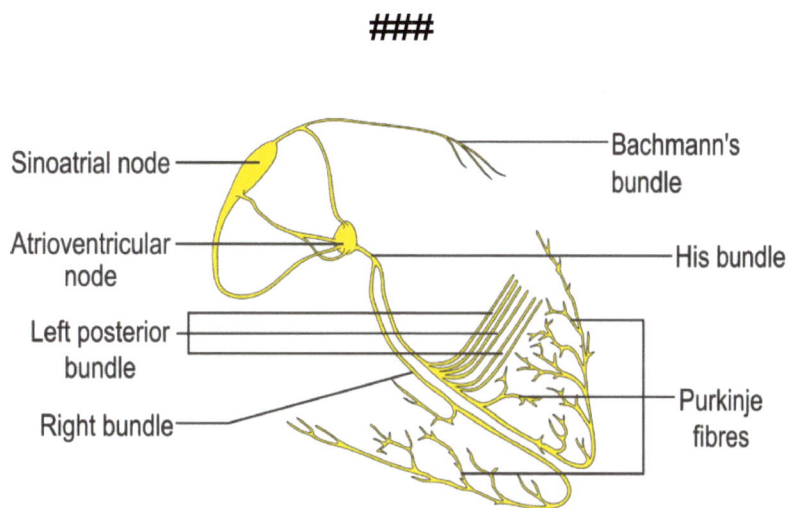

Figure 3.6 Electrical Conduction System of the Heart. Cardiac impulses are initiated at the sinoatrial (SA) node. The left and right bundle branches can be seen leaving the atrioventricular node.

I. Basic Anatomy and Physiology

- The cardiac electrical system has two bundle branches: right and left.
- The bundle branches help to regulate rhythm, and coordinate pumping action of the heart.
  - The bundle branches spread the cardiac electrical impulses evenly across the ventricles, so that when the ventricles contract to eject blood out of the heart, they do so in a coordinated and efficient fashion.

- In BBB, one of the bundle branches is no longer conducting electrical impulses normally because it has become blocked due to disease or damage.
  - BBB may also be incomplete, but these are an incidental finding and usually produce no symptoms.
- The contraction of one ventricle (the one with bundle branch block) occurs slightly after the contraction of the other.
- **RBBB**: right bundle branch no longer conducts electricity
  - Impulse enters the ventricles using only the left bundle branch (first contraction)
  - Then, from the left ventricle, the electrical impulse finally makes its way to the right ventricle (second contraction).
- **LBBB**: left bundle branch no longer conducts electricity
  - Impulse enters the ventricles using only the right bundle branch (first contraction)
  - Then, from the right ventricle, impulse goes to the left ventricle (second contraction).
- With either type of BBB, the QRS complex on the EKG is wider than normal.

II. Clinical Signs and Symptoms

- May have no symptoms (asymptomatic)
- Lightheadedness
- Fainting (syncope)
- Pounding in chest (palpitations)
- Slow or irregular heartbeats
- Shortness of breath
- Difficulty in exercising, because not enough blood is pumped throughout the body
- Presyncope: a feeling that one is about to faint
- LBBB may cause fatigue
- Exercise intolerance

III. Diagnostic Work-up

- Thorough history
- Heart sound assessment
  - Diminished first heart sound and split-second sound with LBBB

- Cardiac enzymes (troponins, creatine kinase, and the erythrocyte sedimentation rate may be useful if myocarditis is suspected).

- Chest X-ray

- An EKG is the most common test for detecting bundle branch block.

  - Certain wave abnormalities may indicate bundle branch block.

  - This test can also determine which bundle branch is affected (the left or right).

  - **Left bundle branch block diagnosis on EKG:**

    ▶ The heart rhythm must be supraventricular (impulse generated in atria) in origin.

    ▶ The QRS duration must be ≥120 msec (>0.12 mm).

    ▶ There should be a QS or rS complex in lead V1.

    ▶ There should be an RsR´ wave in lead V6.

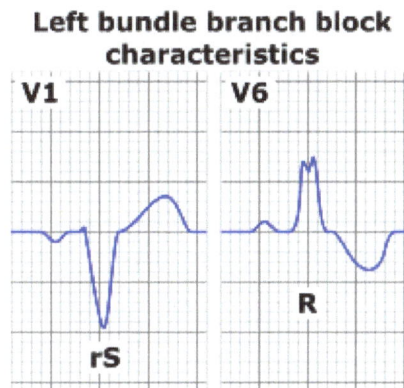

Figure 3.7 EKG of Left Bundle Branch Block.

  - **Right bundle branch block diagnosis on EKG:**

    ▶ The heart rhythm must originate above the ventricles (SA node, atria or AV node) to activate the conduction system at the correct point.

    ▶ The QRS duration must be more than 100 msec (incomplete block) or >120 msec (0.12mm) (complete block).

    ▶ There should be a terminal R wave in lead V1 (e.g., R, rR´, rsR´, rSR´, or qR).

    ▶ There should be a slurred S wave in leads I and V6.

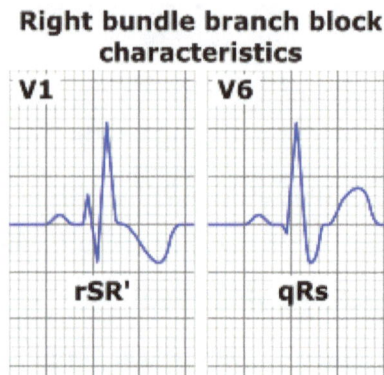

Figure 3.8 EKG of Right Bundle Branch Block.

- ○ **Left *and* right BBB diagnosis on EKG:**

  - ▶ The T wave should be deflected opposite the terminal (last) deflection of the QRS complex. (If the QRS peaks upright, the T wave should dip downwards.)

  - ▶ This is known as appropriate T wave discordance with bundle branch block. A concordant T wave may suggest ischemia or myocardial infarction

- ● Holter tape: a portable device, worn under clothing, which records electrical activity of the heart while the patient goes about normal activities for one or two days. A button is pressed if symptoms are felt, recording the rhythms that were present at that moment.

- ● Echocardiogram: an ultrasound scan that allows the doctor to see the heart muscles and valves.

- ● Electrophysiology test: tiny electrical shocks are used to determine the cause or location of the abnormal rhythm.

- ● Tilt-table test: the patient is placed on a tilt table bed that changes his or her position. This test may sometimes provoke abnormal heartbeats (arrhythmia).

IV. Treatment

- ● The majority of patients with BBB are symptom-free and do not require treatment.

- ● There's no specific treatment for BBB, but the condition indicates the presence of an underlying cardiovascular disease that should be treated.

- ● The main complications of BBB are slow heart rate and fainting; these may require insertion of a pacemaker.

- ● Treat underlying cause if known, and associated conditions:

  - ○ Myocardial infarction

  - ○ Elevated digitalis levels

○ High blood pressure

○ Heart failure

○ Electrolyte abnormalities

● Because heart block affects the electrical activity of the heart, it may be more difficult to quickly diagnose other heart conditions, especially heart attacks.

● New-onset LBBB may be associated with acute MI; look for signs of STEMI, as well.

● Patients having a heart attack should be treated with an anti-ischemic regimen like streptokinase or tissue plasminogen activator (tPA).

○ These drugs dissolve blood clots and improve blood flow to the heart.

○ These medications also carry a risk of bleeding, therefore hospitalization is required.

○ Patients with BBB that involves a heart attack require medications given in an emergency situation; i.e., while en route to a hospital capable of providing cardiology services such as interventional heart catheterization and open heart surgery.

● Current medications should be evaluated and dosages of blocking agents reduced or discontinued to restore electrical conduction.

● Patients with BBB and obvious 1st-degree atrioventricular (AV) block (PR interval >300 msec), those with severe bradycardia, or those believed to be at risk of progression to higher-degree block may be considered for insertion of a dual-chamber pacemaker.

● Medications

○ Atropine: an anticholinergic drug used to increase the heart rate. Adult dose is 0.3–1.2 mg every 4–6 hours (monitor heart rate) *plus*

○ Isoproterenol: a sympathomimetic drug used to increase blood pressure. For adults:

▶ Initial intramuscular dose is 0.2 mg (1 mL) of undiluted 1:5000 solution; then 0.02–1 mg (0.1–5 mL) of undiluted 1:5000 solution.

▶ Intravenous (IV) dilute 1 mL of the 1:5000 solution (0.2mg) to 10 mL with NaCL or D5W (5% dextrose in water).

▷ The initial dose should be 0.02–0.06 mg (1–3 mL) of diluted solution; then, 0.01 –0.2 mg (0.5–10 mL of diluted solution) can be used prior to insertion of pacemaker.

● For information on types of atrioventricular node blocks (1st, 2nd, 3rd degree), EKGs, and treatments, see "Sinus Node Dysfunction and Atrioventricular Block" section in Chapter 3.

● Complete heart block is considered an emergency:

○ Prepare transcutaneous or other pacing equipment and monitor for decompensation (failure of the heart to maintain adequate circulation, marked by labored breathing, engorged blood vessels, and edema).

○ Prepare and provide airway, breathing, and compression support as needed.

○ Except in AV block caused by medications that can be withdrawn, or treatable infections, most patients with complete block will need a pacemaker, or implantable defibrillator.

References

12-Lead ECG Variants, Mimics and Advanced Skills. CardioNursing.
    www.cardionursing.com/wp-content/uploads/2012/04/ECG-Variants-and-Myocardial-Mimics.pdf

BMJ Best Practice.
    bestpractice.bmj.com/best-practice/monograph/728/treatment/step-by-step.html

Budzikowski, Adam S. Third-Degree Atrioventricular Block Treatment and Management. Medscape.
    emedicine.medscape.com/article/162007-treatment#aw2aab6b6b1aa

Bundle Branch Block. About Health. heartdisease.about.com/cs/arrhythmias/a/BBB_2.htm

Bundle Branch Block. Mayo Clinic. www.mayoclinic.com/health/bundle-branch-block/DS00693

Mitchell, L. Brent. Heart Block. Merck Manuals.
    www.merckmanuals.com/professional/cardiovascular-disorders/arrhythmias-and-conduction
    -disorders/bundle-branch-and-fascicular-block

What Is Heart Block? Medical News Today. www.medicalnewstoday.com/articles/180986.php

Figure 3.6 Electrical Conduction System of the Heart. Source: Madhero88 / Wikimedia Commons / CC-BY-SA-3.0. Image at
    commons.wikimedia.org/wiki/File:ConductionsystemoftheheartwithouttheHeart.png

Figure 3.7 EKG of Left Bundle Branch Block. Source: A. Rad / Wikimedia Commons / CC-BY-SA-3.0 / GNU Free Documentation License. Image at
    commons.wikimedia.org/wiki/File:Left_bundle_branch_block_ECG_characteristics.png

Figure 3.8 EKG of Right Bundle Branch Block. Source: A. Rad / Wikimedia Commons / CC-BY-SA-3.0 / GNU Free Documentation License. Image at
    commons.wikimedia.org/wiki/File:Right_bundle_branch_block_ECG_characteristics.png

Supraventricular Tachycardia (SVT)
By Dawn Johnston and Marian M. Houtman

Introduction

- Supraventricular tachycardia (SVT) is an abnormal, rapid heart rhythm that may be sustained or may abruptly start and stop.

- A rhythm that is observed to repeatedly start and stop is called paroxysmal.

- SVT is usually a rhythm of greater than 150 beats per minute.

- SVT can occur in people of all ages and health conditions.

I. Basic Anatomy and Physiology

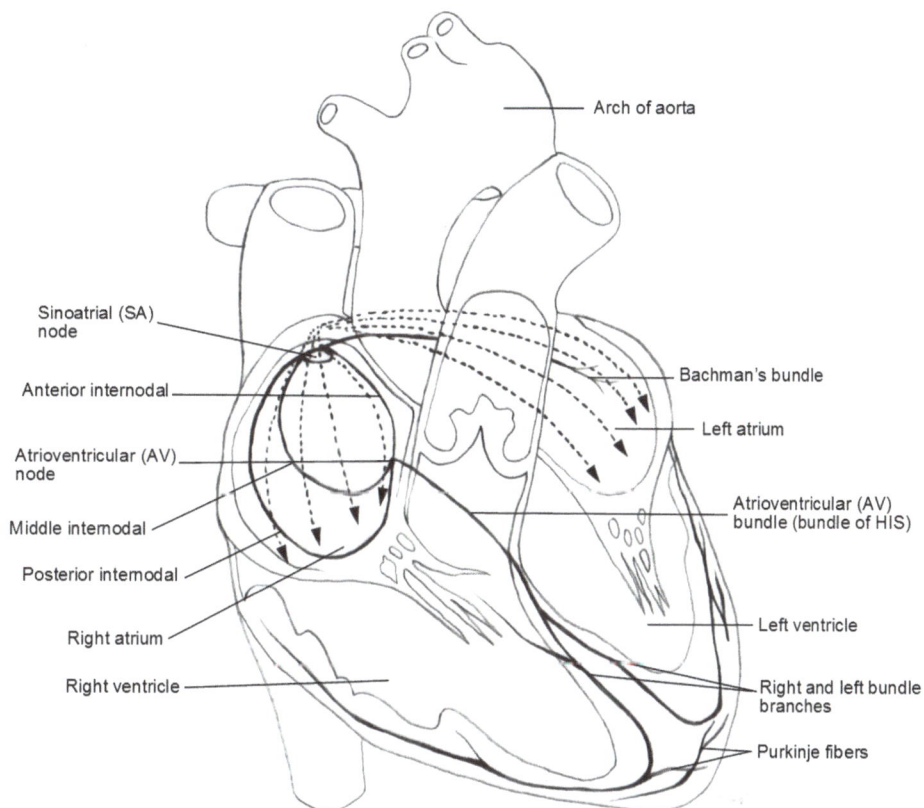

Figure 3.9 Normal Conduction of Impulses through the Heart. These impulses generate adequate contraction of atria and ventricles. In SVT, additional conduction pathways generate many rapid-fire signals that rapidly accelerate the heart rate and impair filling time.

- The initiation and maintenance of SVT happens in the atria and AV node.
- There are multiple types of SVT but all are generated by the sudden activation of additional circuits that bypass the regular conduction of the heart:
  - Accessory pathways
  - Re-entry circuits
- These rapidly firing signals generate a rapid, narrow-complex rhythm on ECG tracings.
- When the heart beats this quickly, it is not able to relax completely to fill with blood for each cardiac contraction and blood pressure often eventually becomes impaired.
- Patients may start to feel dizzy and become unstable.
- SVT can be triggered by:
  - Premature atrial contractions (PACs)
  - Premature ventricular contractions (PVCs)
  - Alcohol intoxication
  - Hyperthyroidism
  - Cardiac disease or prior heart surgery
  - Pneumonia or chronic lung disease
  - Digoxin toxicity
  - Stimulants like caffeine or drugs
- Common types of SVT
  - Most SVTs are regular, narrow-complex without other outstanding ECG features.
  - Wolff–Parkinson–White syndrome is an inherited SVT that can lead to sudden cardiac death, even in young people.
  - SVT with aberrancy (cardiac conduction through abnormal pathways)
    - If a bundle branch block (BBB) is present, impulses are slowed and the rhythm may appear to be wide-complex ventricular tachycardia.
    - Up to 20% of SVTs may have this presentation.

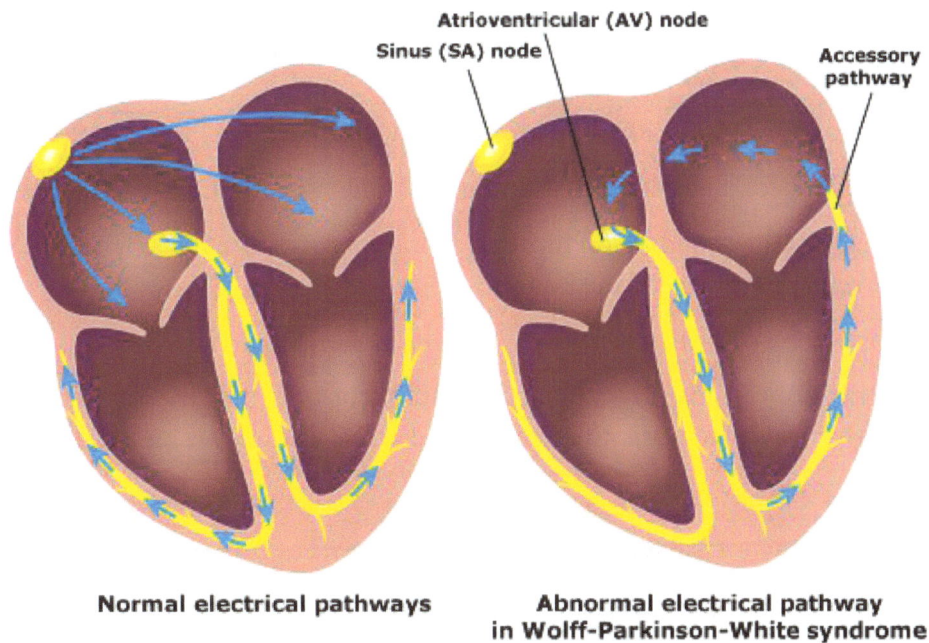

Figure 3.10 Normal Electrical Pathways and Wolff–Parkinson–White Abnormal Conduction Pathway.

II. Clinical Signs and Symptoms

- Patients may be asymptomatic or have palpitations and anxiety.

- Symptoms can come on suddenly and may go away without treatment.

- Stress, exercise and emotions can cause a normal, physiological increase in heart rate, but may also (rarely) bring on SVT.

- SVT episodes can last from a few minutes to 1 or 2 days and sometimes persist until treatment is administered.

- The rapid beating of the heart during SVT can make the heart a less effective pump, decreasing cardiac output and blood pressure.

- Patients may become hemodynamically unstable.

- The following symptoms are typical with a rapid pulse of 150–270 or more beats per minute:
  - Pounding heart
  - Shortness of breath
  - Chest pain
  - Rapid breathing
  - Dizziness or loss of consciousness (serious cases)

○ Numbness in various parts of body

III. Diagnostic Work-up

- Electrocardiogram (ECG/EKG) will be diagnostic for SVT (see Figure 3.11)

- In addition, look for signs of Wolff–Parkinson–White (see Figure 3.12)

- If an SVT has cardiac conduction through abnormal pathways, it can have wide QRS that looks like ventricular tachycardia (VT).

  ○ This is called SVT with aberrancy.

- If not alleviated by standard treatment or if repeat episodes occur, electrophysiology studies may be performed to help identify treatable abnormalities to prevent recurrence.

- Blood tests

  ○ Electrolytes: abnormal levels may contribute to SVT

  ○ Complete blood count: anemia may contribute to SVT or ischemia

  ○ Digoxin level: toxicity can cause paroxysmal SVT

  ○ Thyroid studies: hyperthyroidism may contribute to SVT

- Chest X-ray may be obtained to assess for enlarged heart or fluid building up in the lungs.

- Echocardiogram and magnetic resonance imaging (MRI) may be used if a congenital heart defect is suspected.

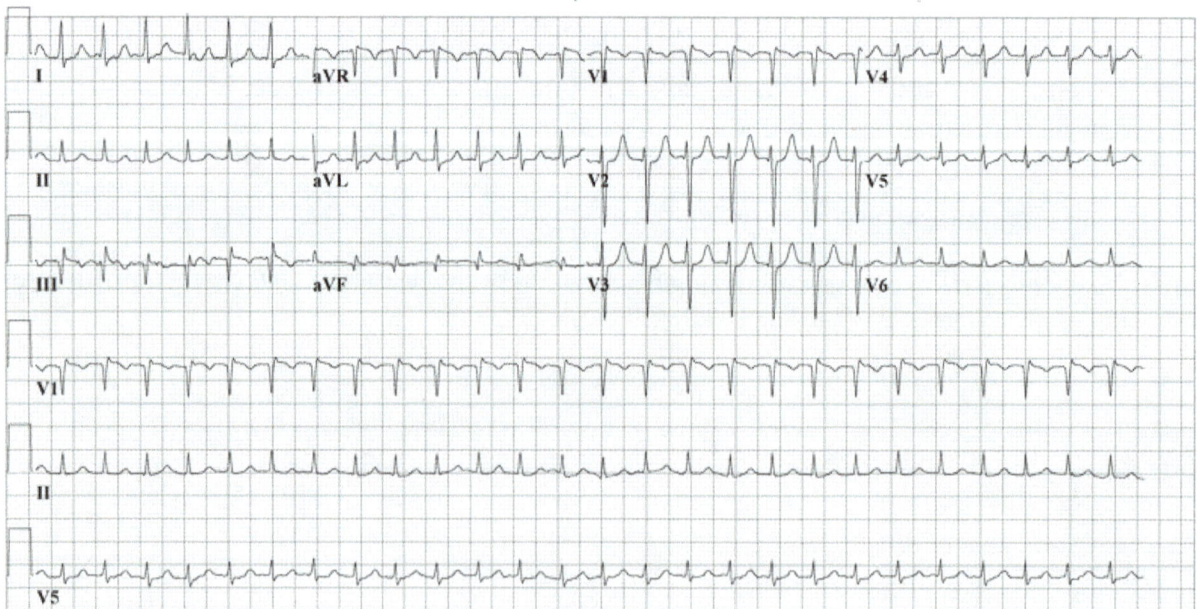

Figure 3.11 Supraventricular Tachycardia (SVT). Most SVTs have narrow QRS complexes and a regular rhythm, as shown in this ECG.

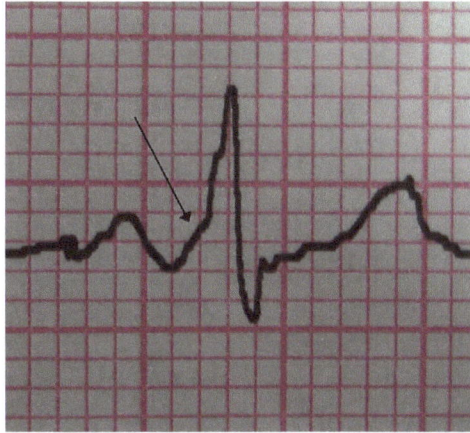

Figure 3.12 Wolff–Parkinson–White, a Type of SVT. The rhythm looks almost identical except for the slurred upstroke of the QRS complex in some leads. This is an inherited defect and should be identified early in life if possible to prevent sudden cardiac death.

IV. Differential Diagnoses

- Sinus tachycardia
- Multifocal atrial tachycardia (MAT)
- Ventricular tachycardia
- Atrial fibrillation
- Atrial flutter

V. Treatment

- SVTs are rarely life-threatening, but episodes can be prevented and treated.
- Rhythms involving the AV node can be stopped by slowing conduction through the AV node.
- Methods of AV blocking:
  - **Physical maneuver (Valsalva)**: activate parasympathetic nervous system or vagal maneuvers
    - Strain as with bowel movement
    - Hold breath
    - Cough
    - Hold nose and blow out
    - Plunge face in cold water

○ **Medication**

▶ Short-term management includes adenosine.

▷ If this works, follow-up by use of diltiazem, verapamil, or metoprolol

○ **Synchronized cardioversion if patient appears symptomatic**

▶ Brief delivery of electrical current depolarizes most cardiac cells, allowing the sinus node to resume normal pacemaker activity.

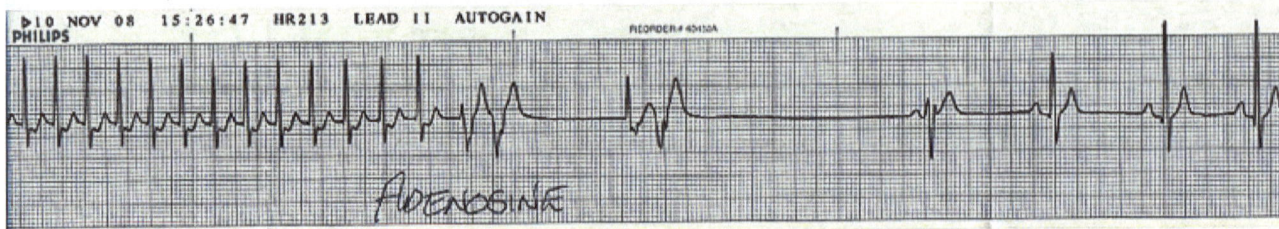

Figure 3.13 SVT Returning to Sinus Rhythm after Adenosine Administered by Rapid IV Push.

Table 3.2 Pharmaceutical Treatment Options for SVT

Drug/Action	Class	Dosage	Contraindications (avoid use in...)
Adenosine Conversion to sinus rhythm	Anti-arrhythmic	6 mg IV over 1–2 seconds; if no response, give 12 mg IV bolus (rapid injection given at one time with a rapid flush)	2nd- or 3rd-degree AV block Sick sinus syndrome without functioning pacemaker Atrial fibrillation or flutter Ventricular tachycardia
Verapamil	Calcium channel blocker	Adults, initial: 5–10 mg (0.075–0.15 mg/kg) as an IV bolus given over 2 minutes (over 3 minutes for older patients); then, if inadequate, 10 mg (0.15 mg/kg) 30 minutes later.	Severe hypotension 2nd- or 3rd-degree AV block Cardiogenic shock Severe congestive heart failure Sick sinus syndrome without functioning pacemaker Severe left ventricular dysfunction

VI. Complications

- Heart attack
- Congestive heart failure
- Syncope (fainting)
- Sudden cardiac death

References

Horenstein, M. Silvana. Junctional Ectopic Tachycardia. Pathophysiology. Medscape.
emedicine.medscape.com/article/898989-overview#a0104

Intravenous Bolus. Medical Dictionary.
medical-dictionary.thefreedictionary.com/intravenous+bolus

Supraventricular Tachycardia. eMedicineHealth.
www.emedicinehealth.com/supraventricular_tachycardia/article_em.htm

Supraventricular Tachycardia. Wikipedia. en.wikipedia.org/wiki/Supraventricular_tachycardia

Figure 3.9 Normal Conduction of Impulses through the Heart. Source: Laura Gajewski, Medical illustrator.

Figure 3.10 Normal Electrical Pathways and Wolff–Parkinson–White Abnormal Conduction Pathway. Source: Tom Luck / Wikimedia Commons / CC-BY-SA-3.0. Image at
commons.wikimedia.org/wiki/File:WPW.jpeg

Figure 3.11 Supraventricular Tachycardia (SVT). Source: Googletrans / Wikimedia Commons / CC-BY-SA-3.0. Image at
commons.wikimedia.org/wiki/File:De-Avnrt_ecg2_(CardioNetworks_ECGpedia).jpg

Figure 3.12 Wolff-Parkinson-White, a Type of SVT. Source: James Heilman, MD / CC-BY-SA-3.0 / GNU Free Documentation License, File:DeltaWave09.JPG. Image at
commons.wikimedia.org/wiki/File:DeltaWave09.JPG

Figure 3.13 SVT Returning to Sinus Rhythm after Adenosine Administered by Rapid IV Push. Source: Biosfear / Wikimedia Commons / CC-BY-SA-3.0. Image at
en.wikipedia.org/wiki/File:Hr_scan.jpg

Multifocal Atrial Tachycardia (MAT)
By Dawn Johnston

Introduction

- Multifocal atrial tachycardia (MAT) is an abnormal rhythm that can originate in the atria of healthy individuals or those with cardiac abnormalities.

- The rhythm is irregular and >100 beats per minute.

- The patient usually has a history of an underlying medical problem; chronic obstructive pulmonary disease (COPD) is the most common associated problem.

- The rhythm is mostly found in elderly males with multiple medical problems.

- MAT itself is seldom life-threatening and usually resolves when the underlying medical ailment is corrected.

- When the rate is variable (<100), the rhythm is sometimes called MAT variant or wandering pacemaker.

I. Basic Physiology

- MAT is caused by several competing sites of atrial impulses generating an irregular rhythm with at least three different-looking P waves.

- MAT may or may not lead to hypotension and instability.

- MAT is most often found in elderly patients with COPD exacerbation, however the mechanism is not well understood.

- MAT is most often a hypoxic complication (involving a deficiency in the amount of oxygen reaching body tissues) that leads to cardiac conduction changes; however, there are other underlying causes.

- MAT is corrected by identifying and treating the underlying condition. These may include:
  - COPD exacerbation
  - Theophylline toxicity
  - Sepsis
  - Electrolyte disturbance
  - Heart failure
  - Coronary artery disease

- ○ Heart valve disease
- ○ Diabetes mellitus
- ○ Azotemia (build-up of urea indicating renal failure)
- ○ Recent surgery
- ○ Pulmonary embolism
- ○ Pneumonia

II. Clinical Signs and Symptoms

- Syncope (fainting)
- Palpitations
- Shortness of breath
- Chest pain
- Lightheadedness

III. Diagnostic Work-up

- Portable anteroposterior (AP) chest X-ray to assess for enlarged heart or other cardiac abnormalities.
- Pulse will be rapid and irregular.
- Patient usually experiences symptoms of whatever disorder is causing the MAT.
- Presentation of 12-lead ECG that demonstrates the signs of MAT (see Figure 3.14)
  - ○ PR intervals are variable.

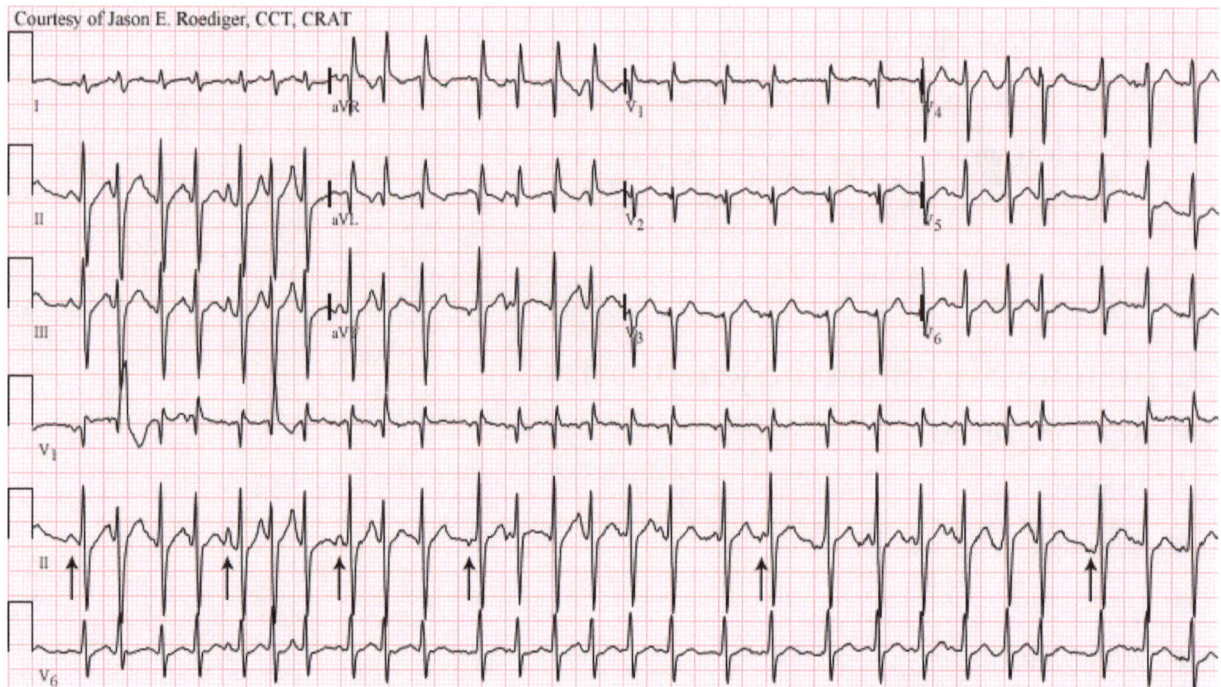

Courtesy of Jason E. Roediger, CCT, CRAT

Figure 3.14 Multifocal Atrial Tachycardia. Note the consistent presence of P waves (see arrows). The constant change in shape indicates that the impulse is generated by different areas in the atria. The result is an irregular rhythm; the heart rate is greater than 100.

- Blood tests are performed based on the suspected underlying disease process:
  - Complete metabolic panel to check for electrolyte imbalance and kidney function.
  - Complete blood count to check for anemia, infection, or clotting problems.
  - Arterial blood gases can assess pulmonary status and need for airway intervention and ventilation strategies.
- Further testing is based on suspected causal pathology, such as:
  - Theophylline level
  - Cardiac enzymes in the presence of abnormal cardiac symptoms

IV. Differential Diagnoses

- Atrial fibrillation
- Atrial flutter
- Supraventricular tachycardia
- Ventricular tachycardia
- Premature atrial contractions

V. Treatment

- Assess for underlying cause of MAT (usually pulmonary) and treat accordingly.
- Stabilize the patient's condition:
  - Sit patient upright if he or she is conscious and short of breath
  - Provide oxygen to keep patient's oxygen saturations within their baseline (>90%).
  - Establish IV, cardiac monitoring, serial blood pressures, and collect list of home medications.
  - Prepare for endotracheal intubation if respiratory failure is imminent.
- Medication options to control heart rate
  - Diltiazem, a calcium channel blocker, is first-line treatment.
    - ▶ 20–40 mg IV bolus, then 10–25 mg/hour infusion
  - Metoprolol, a beta-blocker, may lower the heart rate.
    - ▶ 25 mg orally every 6 hours
  - Magnesium sulfate can lower heart rate quickly if hypokalemia (low potassium) is present.
    - ▶ 2 g IV over 1 minute, then 2 g/hour infusion over 5 hours
    - ▶ After the administration of potassium or magnesium, a slow heart rate due to hypokalemia will resolve.
  - Amiodarone, an antiarrhythmic, can convert MAT to sinus rhythm.
    - ▶ 300 mg by mouth 3 times a day or 450–1500 mg IV over 2–24 hours
- Persistent cases of MAT may be treated with:
  - Radiofrequency ablation (a minimally invasive procedure) and/or
  - Pacemaker placement

VI. Complications

- Stroke from development of blood clots in the atria
- Pulmonary embolism (PE), a condition in which one or more arteries in the lungs become blocked by a blood clot
- Heart attack

References

Budzikowski, Adam S. Atrial Tachycardia. Medscape. emedicine.medscape.com/article/151456-overview

Tandon, Neeraj. Multifocal Atrial Tachycardia. Medscape. emedicine.medscape.com/article/155825-overview

Figure 3.14 Multifocal Atrial Tachycardia. Source: Jer5150 / Wikimedia Commons / CC-BY-SA-3.0. Image at commons.wikimedia.org/wiki/File:Multifocal_atrial_tachycardia_-_MAT.png

Atrial Fibrillation
By Marian M. Houtman

Introduction

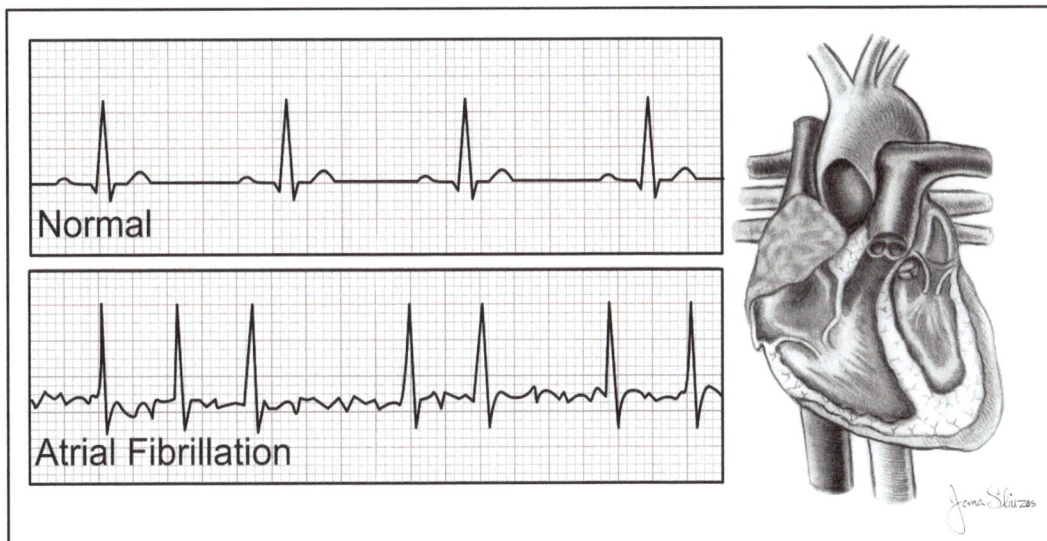

Figure 3.15 Normal Sinus Rhythm and Atrial Fibrillation.

- Atrial fibrillation (A-fib) is an irregular heart rhythm that can lead to stroke if untreated.

- Persistent, new onset A-fib without symptoms requires attempted synchronized conversion to sinus rhythm, but the patient is preferably anticoagulated first.

- If A-fib accelerates to >100 beats/minute, this is called A-fib with a rapid ventricular response (RVR); it may lead to heart failure if the rate is not controlled.

- A-fib with RVR is considered a medical emergency; the patient may be cardioverted (returned to normal rhythm through a medical procedure or administration of drugs) immediately if unstable.

- Risk for developing A-fib increases with age.

- A heart attack may cause A-fib.

- Most patients diagnosed with A-fib notice symptoms but do not suffer harm from the rhythm.

- If untreated, complications can occur, including:

  ○ Blood clots

○ Strokes

○ Heart failure

● A person with A-fib is five to seven times as likely to have a stroke than the general population.

I. Basic Anatomy and Physiology

● Atrial fibrillation begins when the atria (upper chambers) of the heart quiver and no longer provide coordinated contractions to assist with cardiac output.

● This creates stagnant blood in the atria, which promotes the development of clots.

● If one of these clots moves into the ventricle and is ejected through the circulation, major complications can occur:

○ Stroke

○ Pulmonary embolism (PE), a condition in which one or more arteries in the lungs become blocked by a blood clot

● Half of blood clots cause stroke (brain attack); the other half travel to and cause complications in other organs, such as the bowel, kidney, and heart.

● If the rate of A-fib accelerates to >100 beats/minute (A-fib with RVR), the rate must be controlled.

○ A-fib greatly reduces the pumping ability of the heart and can lead to heart failure.

● A-fib may be paroxysmal (intermittent), persistent, or permanent:

○ **Paroxysmal** or intermittent, where the atrial fibrillation starts and stops spontaneously on its own.

▶ Episodes may last anywhere from seconds to days.

○ **Persistent** or occurring in episodes; does not convert back to sinus rhythm spontaneously and patient may become unstable.

▶ Medical treatment or cardioversion (electrical treatment) is required to end the episode.

○ **Permanent** or when the heart is always in atrial fibrillation.

▶ Conversion back to sinus rhythm is not possible or not appropriate for medical reasons.

▶ The rate may be reduced by medications, and patients take anti-clotting medication for life.

● A-fib may exist without underlying heart disease, and is called "lone A-fib."

○ Occurs most commonly in younger people

- ○ May be associated with any of the following:
  - ▶ Hyperthyroidism
  - ▶ Pulmonary embolism
  - ▶ Pneumonia
  - ▶ Excessive alcohol use
  - ▶ Emotional stress
- ● A-fib *with* some underlying cardiac condition is more common, and is called "secondary atrial fibrillation." It may be secondary to any of the following:
  - ○ Heart valve disease
  - ○ Enlargement of left ventricular walls (hypertrophy)
  - ○ Coronary heart disease (coronary artery disease): fatty deposits inside the arteries cause blockages or narrowing of the arteries, interrupting oxygen delivery to the heart muscle (ischemia).
  - ○ High blood pressure
  - ○ Disease of the heart muscle (cardiomyopathy), leading to congestive heart failure
  - ○ Sick sinus syndrome: sinoatrial node stops producing electrical impulses properly.
  - ○ Pericarditis: inflammation of the sack around the heart
  - ○ Myocarditis: inflammation of the heart muscle
  - ○ Advancing age: risk increases beginning at age 40
  - ○ May occur following heart surgery, and resolve a few days after surgery

II. Clinical Signs and Symptoms

- ● No symptoms (asymptomatic) *or*
- ● Sensation of a forceful heart beat (most common with intermittent A-fib)
- ● An irregular flutter in chest
- ● Lightheadedness, faint feeling
- ● Weakness, fatigue
- ● Shortness of breath
- ● Chest pain, angina
- ● Signs indicating life-threatening A-fib:
  - ○ Shortness of breath
  - ○ Low blood pressure

     ○ Uncontrolled chest pain

● Patients in A-fib with RVR, hypotension, severe uncontrolled chest pain, and other signs of shock or ischemia require immediate cardioversion (see Treatment section).

III. Diagnostic Work-up

● Get a complete medical history to assess for risk factors that may complicate treatment or outcomes.

● Physical exam should include an assessment of how well the patient is tolerating the rhythm, including lung sounds, and checking vital signs and other markers of hemodynamic status.

     ○ Obtain a baseline neurologic assessment; prior stroke may make new stroke difficult to determine.

     ○ Other assessment points that may indicate heart failure:

          ▶ Hepatomegaly (enlarged liver)

          ▶ Swelling in the legs

          ▶ Ascites (swelling of the abdomen)

● Chest X-ray should be obtained to assess for an enlarged heart or pulmonary edema.

● Conduct a 12-lead electrocardiogram (EKG/ECG); A-fib characteristics include:

     ○ Irregular rhythm

     ○ Missing P waves

     ○ Often, but not always, the heart rate is >100.

     ○ Chaotic, fibrillation waves at baseline

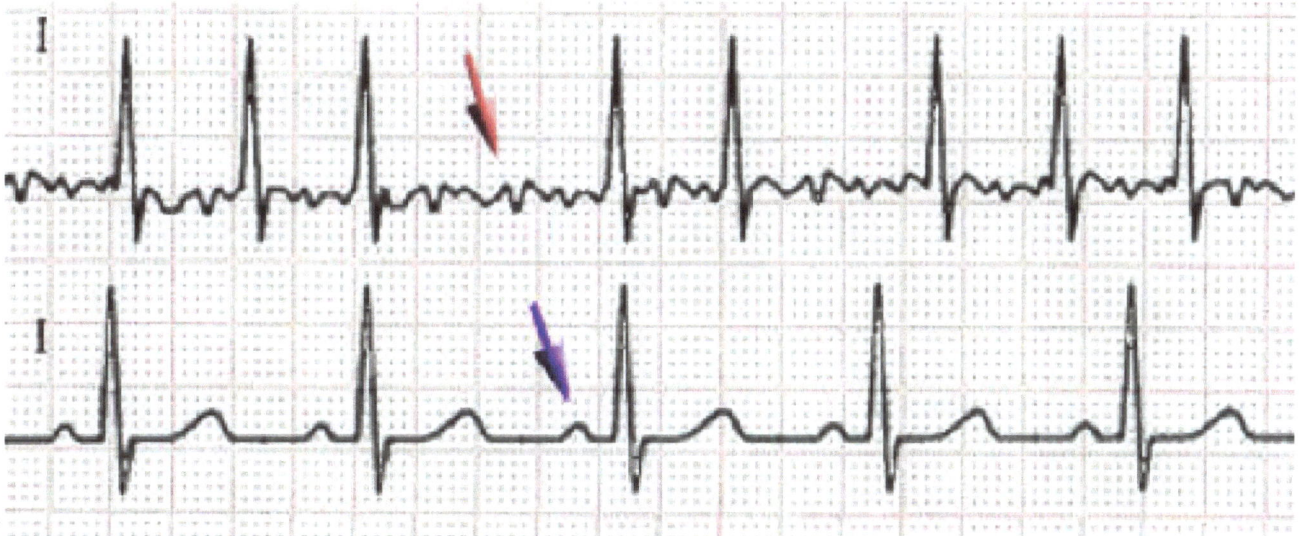

Figure 3.16 EKG Readout of Atrial Fibrillation (top) and Normal Sinus Rhythm (bottom). The purple arrow indicates a P wave in normal sinus rhythm, which is missing/unclear in atrial fibrillation. Instead, irregular fibrillation waves can be seen.

IV. Differential Diagnoses

- Atrial flutter
- Atrial tachycardia
- Supraventricular tachycardia (SVT)
- Wolff–Parkinson–White syndrome (WPW)
- Multifocal atrial tachycardia (MAT)

V. Treatment

- Treatment goals are to slow the heart rate and restore normal rhythm, while providing anti-coagulation medication to avoid blood clots and stroke.
  - Patients who are hypotensive/unstable from A-fib require immediate synchronized cardioversion at 120–200 joules per advanced cardiovascular life support (ACLS) guidelines (biphasic monitor.)
- For patients with A-fib less than 48 hours in duration, synchronized cardioversion may be attempted without anticoagulation.
- When A-fib persists longer than 48 hours, several days or weeks of adequate anticoagulation must be provided before cardioversion is attempted, in order to prevent stroke.
  - As a faster, more practical alternative, IV heparin can be provided and a transesophageal

echocardiography (TEE) performed to document absence of thrombus (a blood clot) prior to cardioversion.

● **Slow the heart rate**

○ If clinical symptoms are present, such as chest pain or shortness of breath, try to decrease the heart rate rapidly with intravenous (IV) medications.

○ Beta blockers and calcium channel blockers (e.g., diltiazem) are first-line agents for rate control.

○ If no symptoms are present, medications may be given by mouth.

○ Patients may require more than one type of oral medication to control the heart rate.

● **Prevent clot formation and stroke**

○ There is an increased risk of stroke in A-fib patients with these co-existing risk factors:

▶ Hypertension

▶ Congestive heart failure

▶ Heart valve abnormalities

▶ Coronary heart disease

▶ Age >65 years

○ Warfarin (brand name Coumadin) is an oral blood-thinning medication used to lower risk of stroke and heart failure in patients awaiting a cardioversion procedure and in those with long-term A-fib.

▶ International normalized ratio (INR) is monitored frequently to confirm therapeutic levels.

▶ Some risk factors like liver disease or hypertension can increase the risk for stroke while on warfarin.

○ Although anticoagulants like warfarin are better at preventing strokes than antiplatelet drugs like aspirin or clopidogrel (brand name Plavix), the latter may be given to some patients who have a low risk of stroke (younger patients with no risk factors) or are unable to take warfarin.

▶ Clopidogrel also prevents clot formation—does not require routine blood testing

○ If it is not advisable or practical to wait days or weeks to achieve therapeutic anticoagulation with warfarin prior to cardioversion, heparin may be administered IV to prevent formation of blood clots in the atria, and cardioversion attempted.

▶ Partial thromboplastin time (PTT) is used to monitor safe levels of anti-coagulation (level should be 50–70 seconds prior to cardioversion attempt).

▶ TEE is used to confirm that there are no clots in the atria, and synchronized cardioversion (a low-energy shock that uses a sensor to deliver electricity that is synchronized with the peak of the QRS complex) is performed.

    ▸ A decision is made later whether the patient needs to be maintained on warfarin.

● **Restore normal rhythm**

    ○ Immediate cardioversion is indicated for patients with new-onset A-fib who present with hypotension and other signs of instability.

    ○ Stable patients with new-onset A-fib should be anticoagulated to a therapeutic level before cardioversion.

        ▸ This may take days or weeks.

        ▸ Rate should be controlled with medications as needed during this time.

        ▸ Normally, warfarin is used to anticoagulate, monitored by INR levels.

        ▸ Alternatively, intravenous heparin may be used, monitored by PTT levels; low-molecular weight heparin is another option.

    ○ About one-half of newly diagnosed A-fib patients will convert to normal rhythm spontaneously in 24–48 hours; however, A-fib often returns.

    ○ Not everyone with A-fib needs to take medication to maintain normal rhythm.

    ○ IV diltiazem or metoprolol are commonly used for A-fib with a rapid ventricular response.

    ○ **Note**: Caution should be exercised in patients with a history of conditions involving wheezing, coughing, or shortness of breath who are given beta-blockers.

    ○ Amiodarone is used as a rate-controlling agent for patients who are intolerant of, or unresponsive to, other agents, such as patients with congestive heart failure who may otherwise not tolerate diltiazem or metoprolol. Caution should be exercised in those who are not receiving anticoagulation, as amiodarone can promote cardioversion.

    ○ Anti-arrhythmia medication is ordered based on how often arrhythmia returns and the symptoms caused. Medication must be carefully tailored to the patient.

    ○ Be aware of unwanted side effects that limit each medication's use.

    ○ *Cardioversion* is a synchronized electrical shock that can convert the patient back to sinus rhythm:

        ▸ More than 90% of people convert to sinus rhythm.

        ▸ It is most successful if the atrial fibrillation is new (hours, days, or a few weeks).

        ▸ Unless the patient is new-onset and unstable (and therefore requires immediate cardioversion), to avoid "throwing a clot" from the atria, he or she should receive a heparin injection first and the PTT should be in a therapeutic range before attempting cardioversion.

        ▸ Prior to cardioversion, a sonogram (TEE) of the heart may be used to determine if any clots are present.

- ▶ A short-term sedative/hypnotic drug may be administered (unless the patient's blood pressure is dangerously low).

  - ▷ The electrical discharge is painful, but sedation is dangerous when hypotension is present.

- ▶ Use patches or paddles and provide a synchronized shock at 120–200 joules, or as per current ACLS guidelines.

● For persistent A-fib that cannot be controlled by medication:

  ○ Radiofrequency ablation is a technique that electrically burns/destroys some of the abnormal conduction pathways in the atria.

  ○ In some patients, most of the atrial electrical activity must be destroyed and an atrial and/or ventricular pacemaker placed to make the heart's ventricles contract in a more normal manner.

Table 3.3 Medication Options for Atrial Fibrillation

Drug Name	Class	Dosage	Use	Special Considerations
Warfarin (Coumadin)	Anti-coagulant	Refer to anticoagulant clinic Monitor prothrombin time and INR during 1st week, or during adjustment period, then monthly. *Initial adult dose:* 5–10 mg/day for 2–4 days, then adjust dose based on PT/INR (INR target should be between 2.0–3.0)	Blood thinner: reduces potential stroke risk	Elderly patients may be more sensitive. Careful monitoring and dosage required when undergoing dental or surgical procedures.
Aspirin	Anti-coagulant	*Myocardial infarction risk, adults:* 160–162.5 mg loading dose, then daily for 30 days. Patients with previous myocardial infarction 75–365 mg per day.	Reduces chance of clot development	Use with caution in the presence of: • Nursing (breastfeeding) • Gastric or peptic ulcers • Mild diabetes • Erosive gastritis • Bleeding tendencies • Cardiac disease • Liver or kidney disease

Drug Name	Class	Dosage	Use	Special Considerations
Clopidogrel (Plavix)	Anti-platelet agent	*Initial*: Single 300 mg loading dose, then 75 mg once daily. Initiate and continue aspirin 75–325 mg, once daily	Reduces chance of clot development	Use with caution: risk of increased bleeding from trauma, surgery, or other pathological conditions.
Diltiazem (Cardizem)	C+ Channel blocker	*A-fib /flutter; paroxysmal supraventricular tachycardia, adults*: 0.25 mg/kg (average 20 mg) given over 2 minutes; then if response is inadequate, a second dose may be given after 15 minutes. The second bolus dose is 35 mg/kg (average 25 mg) given over 2 minutes. Subsequent doses should be individualized.	Controls heart rate in the acute setting	Use of the injectable form is not recommended in newborns. Geriatric patients may be more sensitive to the usual adult dose.
Metoprolol (Lopressor, Toprol XL)	Beta-adrenergic blocking agent	*Angina*: Initially, 100 mg/day in a single dose. Dose may be increased slowly, at weekly intervals until optimal effect or pronounced slowing of heart rate is achieved.	Beta-1 blocking at low dose, Beta-2 blocked at high dose	Dosage has not been established in children. Use with caution if patient has impaired liver function or is nursing.

Drug Name	Class	Dosage	Use	Special Considerations
Amiodarone (Cardarone, Pacerone)	Anti-arrhythmic	If possible, administer in hospital by physician trained in life-threatening arrhythmias. *Loading dose, rapid:* 150 mg over first 10 minutes; then slow loading dose: 360 mg after the next 6 hours (1 mg/minute). *Maintenance dose:* 540 mg over the remaining 18 hours (0.5 mg/minutes). After the first 24 hours, continue maintenance infusion rate of 0.5 mg/minute. This may be continued with monitoring for 2–3 weeks.	Controls rhythm This is a 1st-line drug for left ventricular hypertrophy and for heart failure. Intravenous amiodarone has been shown to slow the ventricular rate and is considered as effective as digoxin.	Safety and effectiveness in children not established. Geriatric patients—especially those with thyroid dysfunction—are more sensitive to this drug than are other adult patients. Monitor carefully in those with left ventricular dysfunction.

VI. Complications

- Stroke
- Pulmonary embolism (PE)
- Heart failure
- Cardiogenic shock

References

Atrial Fibrillation. Cleveland Clinic.
  www.clevelandclinicmeded.com/medicalpubs/diseasemanagement/cardiology/atrial-fibrillation/

Atrial Fibrillation. eMedicineHealth.
  www.emedicinehealth.com/atrial_fibrillation/page8_em.htm

Cardiovascular Center Pocket Guide. University of Michigan.
  www.med.umich.edu/cvc/pocketguides/ami.pdf

Lip, Gregory Y.H. Prevention of Cardiovascular Morbidity Associated with Atrial Fibrillation. Medscape.
  www.medscape.org/viewarticle/708955

New Stroke Risk Factors for Those with Atrial Fibrillation. StopAfig.org.
  www.stopafib.org/newsitem.cfm/NEWSID/220?REFCODE=GooglePPC&Q=chads2

Rosenthal, Lawrence. Atrial Fibrillation: Practice Essentials. Medscape.
  emedicine.medscape.com/article/151066-overview

Spratto, George R., and Woods, Adrienne L. (2004). *PDR Nurse's Drug Handbook, 2004 Edition.* Montvale, NJ: PDR Network.

Figure 3.15 Normal Sinus Rhythm and Atrial Fibrillation. Source: Jana Sliuzas, Medical illustrator.

Figure 3.16 EKG Readout of Atrial Fibrillation (top) and Normal Sinus Rhythm (bottom). Source: J. Heuser / Wikimedia / CC-BY-SA-3.0 / GNU Free Documentation License. Image at
  commons.wikimedia.org/wiki/File:Afib_ecg.jpg

Atrial Flutter

By Marian M. Houtman

Introduction

- Atrial flutter is an abnormality of the heart rhythm, resulting in a rapid and sometimes irregular heartbeat.

- Treatment for atrial flutter is similar to treatment for atrial fibrillation; however, heart rate control is often more difficult to achieve in atrial flutter.

- Atrial flutter can come and go (paroxysmal). More often, atrial flutter lasts for days to weeks (persistent).

- With proper treatment, atrial flutter is rarely life-threatening.

I. Basic Anatomy and Physiology

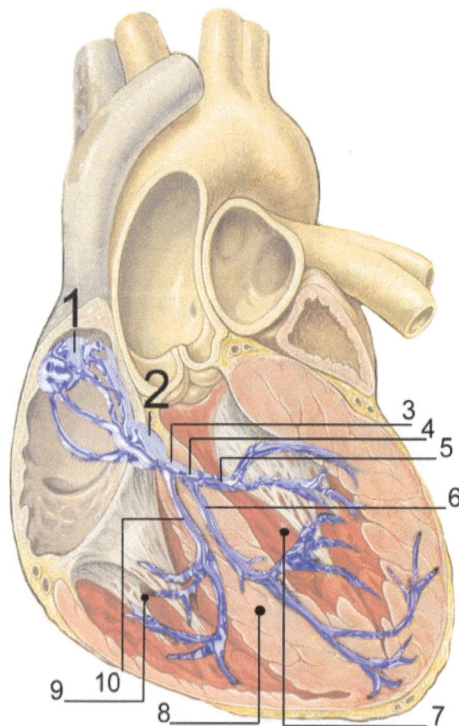

Figure 3.17 Electrical Conduction System of the Heart. Key structures are: **1.** Sinoatrial node (SA), **2.** Atrioventricular node (AV), **3.** Bundle of His, **4.** Bundle branch, **5.** Left posterior fascicle, **6.** Left-anterior fascicle, **7.** Left ventricle, **8.** Ventricular septum, **9.** Right ventricle, **10.** Right bundle branch.

- The abnormal path of the impulses makes the atria contract very rapidly, typically about 250–350 beats per minute.

- The heart beats in a fast, regular rhythm; typically, the ventricular rate is 150 beats/min.

- Main danger: the heart does not pump blood well when it is beating too rapidly.

- When blood is not pumped well, vital organs, such as the heart and brain, may not get enough oxygen from the blood.

- The causes of atrial flutter are primarily connected with conditions and diseases of the heart, including:

  ○ Lack of blood/oxygen to the heart, which can cause hardening of the arteries and heart attack

  ○ High blood pressure

  ○ Disease of heart muscle associated with failure to pump blood

  ○ Abnormality of the heart valves, especially the mitral valve

  ○ Abnormalities of the heart—either congenital (present from birth) or resulting from surgery

  ○ Abnormally enlarged chamber(s) of the heart (hypertrophy)

- Disease elsewhere in the body also is linked to atrial flutter.

  ○ Overactive thyroid gland

  ○ Blood clot to the lungs (pulmonary embolism, or PE)

  ○ Chronic obstructive pulmonary disease (COPD), long-term lung diseases or emphysema, which lowers the amount of oxygen in the blood.

- Consuming the following substances may cause changes in the electrical system of the heart:

  ○ Alcohol

  ○ Caffeine

  ○ Stimulants, such as diet pills, cold medicines, and cocaine

II. Clinical Signs and Symptoms

- Rapid pounding in the chest (palpitations)

- Shortness of breath

- Anxiety

- Weakness

- Some symptoms experienced by patients with underlying heart disease:

  ○ Chest or heart pain (angina)

○ Feeling faint or lightheaded

○ Fainting (syncope)

III. Diagnostic Work-up

- Electrocardiogram (EKG/ECG) shows an atrial flutter saw-tooth appearance

    ○ Atrial flutter waves, known as F waves, can be observed.

    ○ F waves are larger than normal P waves.

    ○ F waves have a saw-toothed form

    ○ Not every F wave results in a QRS complex

- If the EKG result is normal, a portable device called a Holter monitor may be used to monitor electrical activity for 24–48 hours; activity may be monitored for a longer period using an event monitor.

    ○ Patient wears the device for a few days while going about normal activities

    ○ Purpose is to obtain documented proof of the arrhythmia

- An echocardiogram is an ultrasound test that uses sound waves to make a picture of the inside of the heart while it is beating.

    ○ Used to identify heart valve problems, to check ventricular function, or to look for blood clots in the atria

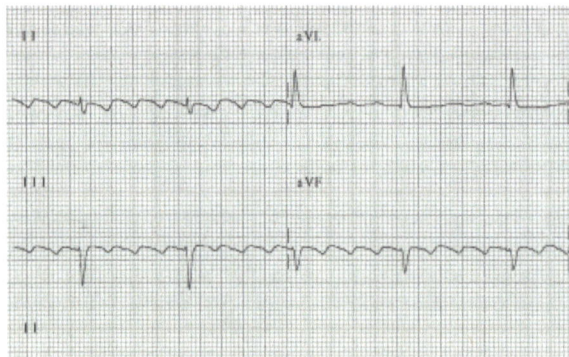

Figure 3.18 EKG of Atrial Flutter.

IV. Treatment

- Most people with atrial flutter have some form of underlying heart disease.

- They require medical treatment to reduce their heart rate and to maintain a normal rhythm.

- The goals of treatment are to control the heart rate and sinus rhythm, to prevent future episodes, and to prevent stroke.
  - Patients who are hypotensive/unstable from atrial flutter require immediate synchronized cardioversion at 50–100 joules per advanced cardiovascular life support (ACLS) guidelines.
- For patients with atrial flutter of less than 48 hours duration, synchronized cardioversion may be attempted without anticoagulation.
- When atrial flutter persists longer than 48 hours, several days or weeks of adequate anticoagulation must be provided before cardioversion is attempted in order to prevent stroke.
  - As a faster, more practical alternative, IV heparin can be provided and a TEE performed to document absence of thrombus prior to cardioversion.
- Control heart rate
  - Direct current (DC) synchronized cardioversion (electric shock)
    - 50–100 joules is recommended per ACLS guidelines for atrial flutter (biphasic monitor).
  - Antiarrhythmic drugs/AV nodal agents
  - Pacemaker
  - Blood pressure medication
  - If patient has NO severe symptoms:
    - In atrial flutter less than 48 hours in duration, attempt to restore normal heart rhythm by electrical synchronized cardioversion as soon as possible.
      - ▷ Sinus rhythm conversion success rate is >95%.
      - ▷ Sedate patient for the procedure (e.g., with etomidate) and begin with 50 joules; less energy is needed than with atrial fibrillation.
    - Refer patient to a hospital for radiofrequency catheter ablation, if possible.
    - If electric shock or ablation are not available, effective, or good options for the patient, consider medication control:
      - ▷ Calcium channel blockers: medications to slow ventricular response
        - ◆ Verapamil
        - ◆ Diltiazem
      - ▷ Digoxin (Lanoxin), a cardiac glucoside that slows heart rate; for patients with poorly functioning left ventricle
      - ▷ Beta blockers: these drugs decrease the heart rate by slowing conduction through the AV node, decreasing the heart's demand for oxygen, and by stabilizing blood pressure

- ◆ Propranolol (Inderal)

- ◆ Metoprolol (Lopressor Toprol XL)

  - ▷ Antiarrhythmics: other antiarrhythmic drugs that can terminate atrial flutter/fibrillation include procainamide, disopyramide, propafenone, sotalol, flecainide, amiodarone, and ibutilide.

  - ▷ Preventing future episodes of atrial flutter involves daily medication to maintain rate/rhythm control and monitoring

- ● Preventing stroke

  - ○ Coexisting conditions, such as coronary heart disease with atrial flutter, significantly increase the risk of stroke.

  - ○ Most people with atrial flutter, including all people older than 65 years, should take a blood-thinning drug called warfarin (Coumadin) to lower this risk.

  - ○ Warfarin blocks the action of certain factors in the blood that promote clotting. In the short term, most patients are put on IV or subcutaneous (administered by injection under the skin) heparin, a drug that immediately decreases the risk of blood clots.

  - ○ A decision is then made whether oral warfarin is needed on a long-term basis.

  - ○ A therapeutic international normalized ratio (INR) should be established for 3 weeks prior to conversion and for at least 4 weeks after conversion to sinus rhythm.

  - ○ People at a lower risk of stroke and those who cannot take warfarin may use aspirin. Aspirin also has side effects, including bleeding, and stomach ulcers.

Table 3.4 Antiarrhythmic Drugs Used in the Treatment of Atrial Flutter

Drug Name	Class	Dosage	Special Considerations
Flecainide (Tambocor)	Anti-arrhythmic	Paroxysmal (at intervals, not consistent/constant) supraventricular tachycardia, paroxysmal A-fib/flutter: 50 mg every 12 hours, dose may then be increased in increments of 50 mg twice a day every 4 days until effective	Control rhythm rather than rate. This is a 1st-line drug for patients without heart disease. Use with caution in the presence of: Sick sinus syndrome Congestive heart failure Myocardial infarction Potassium disturbances Patients with permanent pacemakers or temporary pacing electrodes Kidney/liver impairment.
Propafenone (Rythmol)	Anti-arrhythmic	*Adults, initial dose*: 150 mg every 8 hours; dose may be increased at a minimum of every 3–4 days to 225 mg every 8 hours, and, if necessary, to 300 mg every 8 hours.	Control rhythm. This is a 1st-line drug for patients without heart disease. Increased risk of death in non-life-threatening arrhythmias. Use with caution during labor/delivery, and if kidney/liver impairment is present. Use not determined in children.

Drug Name	Class	Dosage	Special Considerations
Sotalol (Betapace)	Anti-arrhythmic	Ventricular arrhythmias *Adult dose*: 80 mg twice/day. The dose may be increased to 240 or 320 mg/day after appropriate evaluation.	Control rhythm. This is a 1st-line drug for patients without heart disease, and for patients with coronary artery disease. Patients with sustained ventricular tachycardia and history of congestive heart failure appear to be at the highest risk for serious proarrhythmia (new arrhythmia or aggravation of pre-existing arrhythmia). Use with caution in the presence of: Bronchitis Emphysema, asthma, sick sinus syndrome Reduced kidney function. Use not established in children.
Amiodarone (Cardarone, Pacerone)	Anti-arrhythmic	If possible, delivered by a trained physician. *Loading dose, rapid*: 150 mg over first 10 minutes, then slow loading dose: 360 mg after the next 6 hours (1 mg/minute). *Maintenance dose*: 540 mg over the remaining 18 hours (0.5 mg/minute). After 1st 24 hours, continue maintenance infusion rate of 0.5 mg/minute. May be continued with monitoring for 2–3 weeks.	Control rhythm. This is a 1st-line drug for left ventricular hypertrophy and for heart failure. Intravenous amiodarone has been shown to slow the ventricular rate and is considered as effective as digoxin. Safety and effectiveness in children not established. Geriatric patients, especially those with thyroid dysfunction, may be more sensitive to this drug. Monitor carefully in those with left ventricular dysfunction.

Drug Name	Class	Dosage	Special Considerations
Adenosine (Adenocard)	Anti-arrhythmic	*Initial dose*: 6 mg IV over 1–2 seconds. If the 1st dose does not reverse the paroxysmal supraventricular tachycardia within 1–2 minutes, 12 mg dose should be given as rapid IV bolus. A 12 mg dose may be repeated a second time, if necessary. Doses greater than 12 mg not recommended.	Adenosine is an antiarrhythmic drug. It works by slowing the electrical conduction in the heart, slowing heart rate, or normalizing heart rhythm. It can be used to *unmask* type I atrial flutter.

Administered in an IV push followed with an IV bolus with flush, adenosine can also be helpful in making the diagnosis of atrial flutter by briefly blocking the AV node. |

Table 3.5 Calcium Channel Blockers, Cardiac Glycosides, and Beta Blockers Used in the Treatment of Atrial Flutter

Drug Name	Class/Action	Dosage	Special Considerations
Verapamil (Calan Isoptin)	Calcium channel blocker; diminishes premature ventricular contractions	Dosage range in digitalized* patients with chronic atrial fibrillation: 240–320 mg/ day in divided doses, 3–4 times/ day.

Supraventricular tachyarrhythmias

Initial dose for adults is 5–10 mg (0.075–0.15 mg/kg) as an IV bolus given over 2 minutes (administered over 3 minutes in older adults); then 10 mg (0.15 mg/kg) 30 minutes later if response is inadequate.

*Digitalized means that patient is given digitalis up to a level that is effective. | Infants age <6 months may not respond to verapamil.

Use with caution in the presence of hypertrophic cardiomyopathy, impaired kidney/ liver and in elderly patients. |

Drug Name	Class/Action	Dosage	Special Considerations
Diltiazem (Cardizem)	C+ channel blocker— heart rate control	A-fib/flutter; paroxysmal supraventricular tachyarrhythmias Initial dose for adults is 0.25 mg/kg (average 20 mg) given over 2 minutes; if response is inadequate, a second dose may be given after 15 minutes. The second bolus dose is 0.35 mg/kg (average 25 mg) given over 2 minutes. After this, doses should be individualized.	Use of the injectable form is not recommended in newborns. Geriatric patients may be more sensitive to the usual adult dose.
Digoxin capsules* (Lanoxin) *Other dosage guidelines apply to digoxin tablets and elixir.	Cardiac glycoside; decreases conductivity of electrical impulses through AV node. Used primarily in patients with heart disease, left ventricular failure.	To achieve **rapid digitalization**, initial adult dose is 0.4–0.6 mg, followed by 0.1–0.3 mg every 6–8 hours until desired effect achieved. For **slow digitalization** in adults, a total of 0.05–0.35 mg/day divided in 2 doses for a period of 7–22 days to reach steady state serum levels.	Check digoxin level when determining cause for atrial flutter (rule out). Use with caution in patients with: • Heart disease with unknown cause • Acute myocarditis • Hypertrophic subaortic stenosis, hypoxic or myxedemic states • Adam–Stokes or carotid sinus syndrome • Cardiac amyloidosis • Cyanotic heart and lung disease, including emphysema and partial heart block
Propranolol (Inderal)	Beta-adrenergic blocking agent with Beta-1 and Beta-2 blocking activity	Arrhythmias 10–30 mg 3–4 times/day, before meals and at bedtime	

Drug Name	Class/Action	Dosage	Special Considerations
Metoprolol (Lopressor, Toprol XL)	Beta-adrenergic blocking agent with Beta-1 and Beta-2 blocking activity	Angina Initially, 100 mg/day in a single dose. Dose may be increased slowly, at weekly intervals until optimal effect or pronounced slowing of heart rate is achieved.	Dosage has not been established In children. Use with caution in patients with impaired kidney function and/or those who are nursing.

###

Table 3.6
Anticoagulant and Antiplatelet Agents Used in the Treatment of Atrial Flutter

Drug Name	Class/Action	Dosage	Special Considerations
Warfarin (Coumadin)	Anticoagulant (blood thinner); reduces potential stroke risk	Refer to anticoagulation clinic. Monitor prothrombin time/international normalized ratio during first week, or during adjustment period, then monthly. Initial adult dose, 5–10 mg/day for 2–4 days; then adjust dose based on prothrombin time or INR.	Elderly patients may be more sensitive. Careful monitoring and dosage required for patients undergoing dental or surgical procedures.
Aspirin	Anticoagulant; reduces chance of clot development	Heart attack risk, *adults:* 160–162.5 mg, loading dose, then daily for 30 days. Previous heart attack 75–365 mg per day.	Use with caution in nursing patients and in the presence of: • Gastric or peptic ulcers • Mild diabetes • Erosive gastritis • Bleeding tendencies • Cardiac disease • Liver or kidney disease

Drug Name	Class/Action	Dosage	Special Considerations
clopidogrel (Plavix)	Antiplatelet agent Reduces chance of clot development	Initially in adults, a single 300 mg loading dose, then 75 mg once daily. Initiate and continue aspirin 75–325 mg once daily	Use with caution in those at risk of increased bleeding from trauma, surgery, or other pathological conditions.

###

V. Complications

- Syncope
- Heart failure
- Cardiogenic shock

VI. Prevention

- A healthy lifestyle may reduce the chance of coronary heart disease, which can lead to atrial flutter.
- "Heart-healthy living" as recommended by the American Heart Association
  - Do not smoke
  - Engage in moderately strenuous physical activity for at least 30 minutes a day
  - Eat nutritious foods that are low in cholesterol and other fats
  - Maintain a healthy weight
  - Control high blood pressure and high cholesterol.

References

Atrial Flutter. eMedicineHealth. www.emedicinehealth.com/atrial_flutter/article_em.htm

Borczuk, Pierre. Emergent Management of Atrial Flutter. Medscape. emedicine.medscape.com/article/757549-overview#a30

Spratto, George R., and Woods, Adrienne L. (2004). *PDR Nurse's Drug Handbook, 2004 Edition.* Montvale, NJ: PDR Network.

Figure 3.17 Electrical Conduction System of the Heart. Source: Patrick Lynch, Carl Jaffe, J. Heuser / Wikimedia Commons / CC-BY-SA-2.5. Image at en.wikipedia.org/wiki/File:RLS_12blauLeg.png

Figure 3.18 EKG of Atrial Flutter. Source: Ksheka / Wikimedia Commons / CC-BY-SA-3.0 / GNU Free Documentation License. Image at en.wikipedia.org/wiki/File:Atrial_flutter_with_4-1_AV_block.png

Wolff–Parkinson–White Syndrome

By Marian M. Houtman

Introduction

- Wolff–Parkinson–White syndrome (WPW) is a condition that is present from birth, involving abnormal conductive tissue between the atria and ventricles.

- WPW is a type of supraventricular tachycardia (SVT) in which the heart beats very fast.

- Dangerous ventricular arrhythmias may develop due to extremely fast conduction across a tract bypassing the AV node, especially if atrial flutter or A-fib develops.

- A small percentage of people with this syndrome (<1%) are at risk for sudden cardiac death.

- All ages, including infants, can experience the symptoms related to WPW syndrome.

- Episodes of a fast heartbeat often first occur in the teenage years or early twenties.

- It is more frequent in males than females; in most cases, episodes of fast heartbeats are not life-threatening, but serious heart problems can occur.

- Common causes or triggers:
  - Coronary heart disease
  - Ischemia
  - Cardiomyopathy
  - Pericarditis
  - Electrolyte disturbances
  - Thyroid disease
  - Anemia (abnormally low number of red blood cells in the blood)

I. Basic Anatomy and Physiology

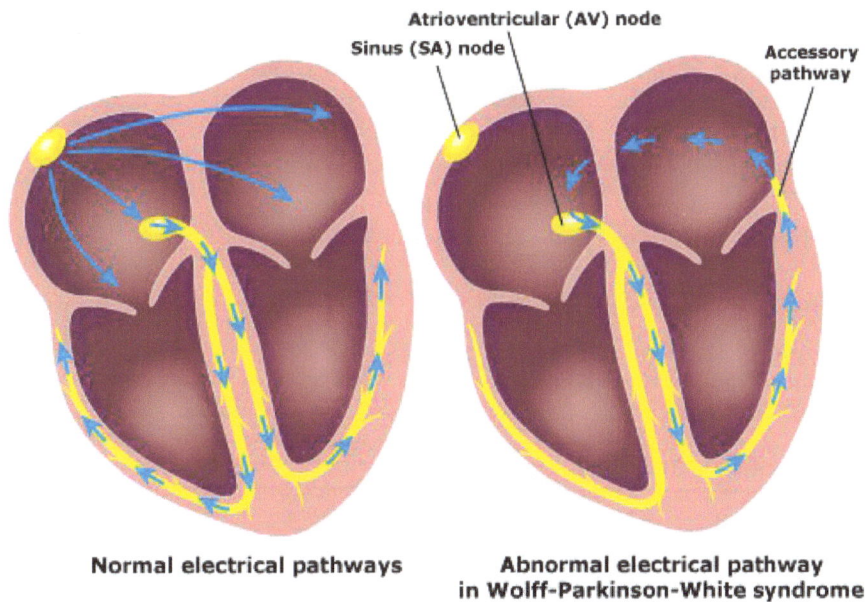

Figure 3.19 Normal Electrical Pathways and Wolff–Parkinson–White Abnormal Conduction Pathway.

II. Clinical Signs and Symptoms

- Classic EKG findings in WPW:
  - Presence of a short PR interval (<120 msecs)
  - A wide QRS complex longer than 120 msecs with a slurred onset of the QRS waveform producing a delta wave in the early part of QRS
  - Secondary ST-T wave changes

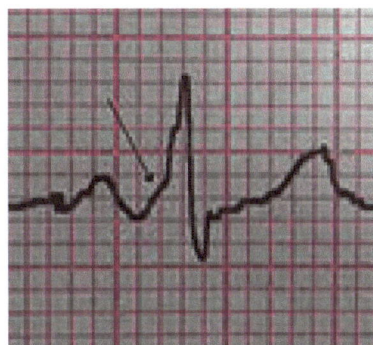

Figure 3.20 Delta Wave (indicated by arrow) Seen in the Beginning of the QRS Complex. This slurred upstroke of the QRS complex is evidence of WPW.

- Symptoms may include:
  - Mild chest discomfort
  - Feeling of a pounding heart, with or without fainting
  - Severe cardiopulmonary compromise or cardiac arrest
- Infants with WPW:
  - May frequently be irritable
  - May not be able to eat, or digest food properly (spitting up, vomiting, screaming)
  - May demonstrate evidence of congestive heart failure
  - May exhibit unusual behavior for 1–2 days
  - Often develop a fever
- Symptoms in children include:
  - Usually report of chest pain (if child is able to talk)
  - Feeling of a pounding heart
  - Breathing difficulty
  - A positive family history of this condition
- Older patients with WPW may have:
  - Sudden onset of a pounding heartbeat
  - Change in tolerance for activity
  - A regular rhythm that may indicate the presence of A-fib
  - WPW that will be found on a routine electrocardiography (EKG/ECG)
  - Light-headedness and near fainting (more common in those with WPW syndrome who have paroxysmal SVT or A-fib, than in those with atrioventricular nodal reentry)
  - Fainting that occurs because of inadequate blood to the brain from rapid ventricular rate

III. Diagnostic Work-up

- Extent of the work-up is determined by the severity of illness.
- If the heart is severely damaged and unable to supply enough blood to organs, or patient is unconscious:
  - In condition caused by WPW rhythm, direct current (DC) cardioversion is indicated.
- Once the patient's blood flow is adequate, laboratory studies to be considered are:
  - Electrolytes with potassium
  - Complete blood count

- ○ Blood urea nitrogen
- ○ Liver function tests
- ○ Thyroid panel
- ○ Magnesium
- ○ Calcium
- ○ Arterial blood gases
- ○ Lactate levels
- ○ Drug screening and drug levels
- Electrocardiographic (EKG/ECG) monitoring and 12-lead EKG
- Thorough history and physical examination
- Echocardiography to rule out cardiomyopathy and congenital heart defect, such as hypertrophic cardiomyopathy.
- Refer for electrophysiologic study if available (done in diagnostic clinic).
- The diagnosis of WPW is typically made with EKG monitoring, and clues from the history and physical examination.
- Evaluate patients with symptomatic tachycardia (supraventricular tachycardia or wide-complex tachycardia) for the presence of pre-excitation (early activation of the ventricles) on 12-lead EKG results, and consider consultation with a cardiac electrophysiologist (a cardiologist with advanced training in heart rhythms).
- Evaluate for the presence of very short refractory periods which put patients at a higher risk of developing symptoms or complications, and poor response to drug therapy. Identify these patients, even if no symptoms are present, and refer for electrophysiologic study and ablation.

IV. Treatment

- **Unstable patient**
  - ○ Cardiac arrest and blood circulation compromise require ABCs (airway, breathing, circulation).
  - ○ Have a defibrillator available and provide appropriate monitoring.
  - ○ If the patient is experiencing a dysrhythmia (disturbance of heart rhythm), provide DC cardioversion.
- **Stable patient**
  - ○ Vagal maneuvers may be attempted (in infants, a bag of ice slurry to the face is very effective; in children, have the patient blow with thumb in mouth, like a trumpet).

- ○ If conservative measures fail, give adenosine.
  - ▶ Do not use if patient has pre-excited A-fib.
  - ▶ Effective in approximately 90% of reentrant narrow-complex tachycardias
  - ▶ Must be administered as a rapid bolus because of its short half-life. Most cases of adenosine failure in this setting are caused by inadequate administration.
  - ▶ A defibrillator must be available in the event that new dysrhythmias emerge, particularly post-adenosine A-fib.
- ○ Considerations:
  - ▶ Procainamide and esmolol for use in resistant cases
  - ▶ Verapamil should not be used if patient is age <1 year due to risk of severe hypotension, severe bradycardia, or heart failure.
  - ▶ Verapamil can also accelerate ventricular rate in A-fib, leading to V-fib.
- ● Ongoing management of WPW is aimed at addressing the underlying cause of the condition through the use of:
  - ○ Radiofrequency ablation
  - ○ Antiarrhythmic drugs to slow conduction through the abnormal pathway
    - ▶ Blocking medications to slow conduction through the AV node
  - ○ Treatment of the triggers that perpetuate the dysrhythmia
    - ▶ Individualized plan for each patient
    - ▶ Individual risk assessment, based on the likely prognosis and on the degree of symptoms the patient experiences.
  - ○ Medication
    - ▶ Beta-blockers
      - ▷ Most common use: supraventricular tachycardia in the presence of pre-excitation
      - ▷ These agents are moderately effective; adverse effects are frequent, but rarely life-threatening, unless patient has a reactive airway disease.
    - ▶ More potent medications (flecainide, propafenone, sotalol, or amiodarone) may have greater effects on abnormal pathway conduction and on refractory period than do beta-blockers and are therefore preferred by some physicians.
    - ▶ Contraindicated medications (avoid use in WPW syndrome):
      - ▷ Digoxin or verapamil may enhance conduction through the abnormal pathway by increasing the time it takes for the AV node to be ready for another stimulation (refractory period).
      - ▷ Digoxin may also decrease the time it takes for the abnormal pathway to be ready

for another stimulation, further enhancing its conduction.

▶ Use class Ic and class III antiarrhythmic medications with caution in WPW syndrome (see Table 3.7).

▷ These agents slow down abnormal pathway conduction, increasing risk of blockage of supraventricular tachycardia. If the patient has a history of A-fib or atrial flutter, an AV nodal blocking medication should also be used.

○ The best long-term plan is to not use drugs at all. All patients who have WPW syndrome with symptoms should be referred for electrophysiologic study, and referred for ablation, if possible. Patients who have abnormal pathway conduction without symptoms, and short refractory periods (<240 msec), are also best treated with ablation.

Table 3.7
Pharmaceutical Treatment Options for Wolff–Parkinson–White Syndrome

Class	Example	Mechanism	Clinical use
Ia Fast channel blockers; affect QRS complex	Quinidine Procainamide Disopyramide	Na+ channel block intermediate association/ dissociation	Ventricular arrhythmias Prevention of paroxysmal recurrent A-fib (triggered by vagal overactivity) Procainamide in WPW syndrome
Ic	Flecainide Propafenone Moricizine	Na+ channel block slow association/ dissociation	Prevents paroxysmal atrial fibrillation Treats recurrent tachyarrhythmias of abnormal conduction system Contraindicated immediately post-myocardial infarction.
II Beta blockers	Propranolol Esmolol Timolol Metoprolol Atenolol Bisoprolol	Beta-blocking Propranolol also shows some class I action	Decreases myocardial infarction mortality Prevents recurrence of tachyarrhythmias

Class	Example	Mechanism	Clinical use
III	Amiodarone Sotalol Ibutilide Dofetilide Dronedarone E-4031	K+ channel blocker Sotalol is also a beta blocker [2]. Amiodarone is a Class III antiarrhythmic drug, but has electrophysiologic characteristics of Class I,II, IV.	In WPW syndrome Sotalol, ventricular tachycardias and atrial fibrillation Ibutilide, atrial flutter and atrial fibrillation
IV Slow channel blocker	Verapamil Diltiazem	Ca+ channel blocker	Prevents recurrence of paroxysmal supraventricular tachycardia Reduces ventricular rate in patients with A-fib

###

V. Patient Education

- Patient education is very important, especially young patients with abnormal EKG results, but no symptoms.

- Periodic follow-up care is necessary.

- Discuss electrophysiologic study and ablation if it is an option for the patient.

- Patients should carry sample EKG in sinus rhythm and a medical identification bracelet.

- If treated with medications, educate patients about the following:

  ○ How to recognize disease recurrence

  ○ How to perform vagal maneuvers, when needed

  ○ Importance of keeping follow-up appointments

  ○ How to identify the adverse effects of antiarrhythmic drugs

  ○ Importance of avoiding competitive sports

- Patients should educate family members, and siblings should be screened for pre-excitation with 12-lead EKG.

References

Antiarrhythmic Agents. Wikipedia. en.wikipedia.org/wiki/Antiarrhythmic_agent

Ellis, Christopher R. Long-Term Antiarrhythmic Therapy. Medscape. emedicine.medscape.com/article/159222-treatment#aw2aab6b6b7aa

Ellis, Christopher R. Wolff-Parkinson-White Syndrome. Medscape. emedicine.medscape.com/article/159222-overview

Intracardic Electrophysiology Study. MedlinePlus. www.nlm.nih.gov/medlineplus/ency/article/003867.htm

Figure 3.19 Normal Electrical Pathways and Wolff–Parkinson–White Abnormal Conduction Pathway. Source: Tom Luck / Wikimedia Commons / CC-BY-SA-3.0. Image at commons.wikimedia.org/wiki/File:WPW.jpeg

Figure 3.20 Delta Wave (indicated by arrow) Seen in the Beginning of the QRS Complex. Source: James Heilman / Wikimedia Commons / CC-BY-SA-3.0 Documentation. Image at en.wikipedia.org/wiki/File:DeltaWave09.JPG

Premature Ventricular Contractions
By Marian M. Houtman

Introduction

- Premature ventricular contractions (PVCs) are extra heartbeats that originate in the ventricles.

- These extra (ectopic) heartbeats occur before the heart's normal conduction is triggered, which causes an interruption in the heart's rhythm.

- A PVC can be observed as a wide, bizarre complex on the monitor or 12-lead ECG.

- PVCs are one of the most common arrhythmias, and can occur in patients with or without heart disease.

- Occasional PVCs are especially common in older people with cardiac disease; infrequent PVCs are generally well-tolerated.

- Frequent PVCs can herald the onset of serious cardiac arrhythmias like ventricular tachycardia, or otherwise indicate a need for intervention.

I. Pathophysiology

- Contraction of the ventricles occurs from an impulse that is generated from a site below the atrioventricular node (AVN).
  - Results from conduction errors and excitability within the heart
- People of African (black) descent and men are at greater risk than the rest of the population.
- Importance of PVCs depends on clinical context:
  - PVCs in young, healthy patients without underlying structural heart disease are usually not associated with any increased rate of mortality (death).
  - PVCs in older patients, in particular those with underlying heart disease, are associated with an increased risk of adverse cardiac events (sustained ventricular dysrhythmias and sudden death).
  - In patients who have had a heart attack, the risk of ventricular arrhythmias and sudden death is related to the complexity and frequency of the PVCs.
  - Frequent PVCs are associated with increased risk of stroke in patients who do not have hypertension (high blood pressure) and diabetes.

- Increased PVC frequency with age is due to the increased prevalence of hypertension and cardiac disease in aging populations.
- Cardiac-related causes of PVCs may include:
  ○ Acute myocardial infarction or lack of blood to heart muscle
  ○ Myocarditis: inflammation of heart muscle
  ○ Cardiomyopathy: diseases of the heart muscle
  ○ Myocardial contusion: bruises or injuries to the heart muscle
  ○ Improper closing of the mitral valve separating the left atrium and left ventricle
- Other causes may include:
  ○ Low oxygen level or high carbon dioxide level in blood
  ○ Medications/substances that affect the sympathetic nervous system (digoxin, tricyclic antidepressants, aminophylline, caffeine)
  ○ Such substances as cocaine, amphetamines, alcohol, and tobacco
  ○ Low magnesium or low potassium levels, high calcium levels

II. Clinical Signs and Symptoms

- Obtain a history from patients (past PVCs, cardiac disease or structural heart disease)
- Identify medications that increase risk of arrhythmias, abnormal potassium or magnesium levels. These substances may also cause PVCs: ephedrine-containing drugs, excessive caffeine, and cocaine.
- PVCs often accompany blood supply/oxygen shortages, and indicate cardiac disease or myocardial infarction; evaluate for chest pain and blood flow changes, such as lightheadedness or fainting.
- Frequent PVCs may cause blood flow problems. Clinically evident hypotension (low blood pressure) is rare, but relative hypotension is not uncommon, particularly in patients with underlying cardiac disease.
- PVCs may produce a weakened or absent pulse, depending on force of contraction.

III. Diagnostic Work-up

- Laboratory studies:
  ○ Serum electrolyte levels, particularly potassium
  ○ Magnesium levels, especially in patients with low potassium
  ○ A drug screen may be helpful in some patients.

○ Drug levels if taking medication with known pro-arrhythmic effects (e.g., digoxin, theophylline)

● Standard 12-lead EKG. Findings may include:

○ Left ventricular hypertrophy

○ Active cardiac ischemia (ST-segment depression or elevation, and/or T-wave inversion)

○ If previous myocardial infarction, Q waves or loss of R waves, bundle branch block

○ Electrolyte abnormalities (taller, more pointed T waves, longer QT)

○ Drug effects (QRS widens, longer QT)

○ PVCs may be premature in relation to the next expected beat of the basic rhythm. The pause after the premature beat is usually a full compensatory pause, which means the R-R interval surrounding the premature beat is equal to double the basic R-R interval.

○ PVCs may appear in a pattern of every other, every third, or every fourth beat.

● Holter 24-hour monitors are useful in counting and characterizing ventricular abnormal beats.

● Echocardiography evaluates percentage of blood leaving the heart each time it contracts, which is helpful in prognosis and in identifying valvular disease or ventricular hypertrophy.

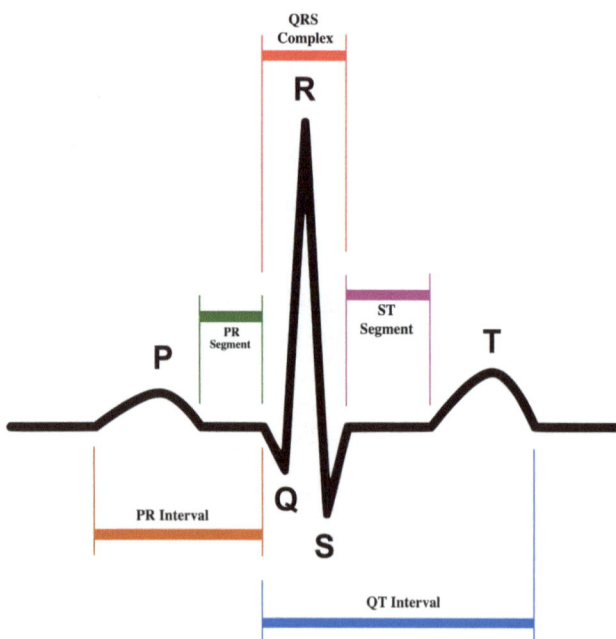

Figure 3.21 Normal Sinus Rhythm.

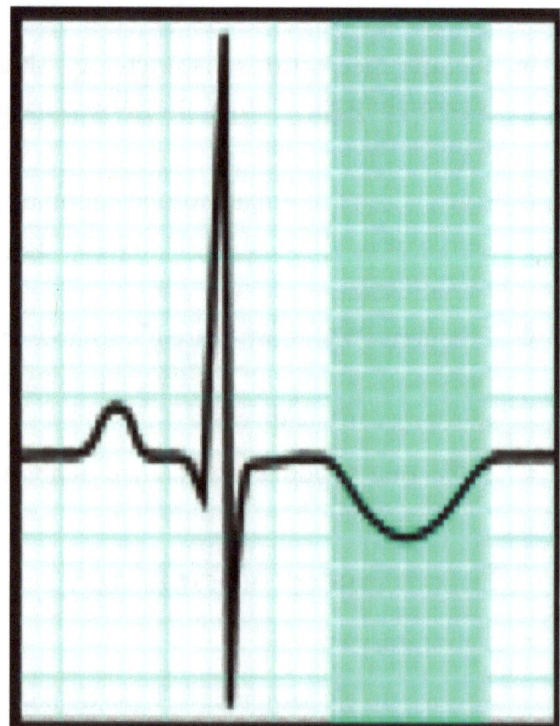

Figure 3.22 Inverted T Wave in Lead V6.

IV. Differential Diagnoses

- Acute coronary syndrome

- Heart attack

- Myocarditis: inflammation of the heart muscle

- Ventricular fibrillation: uncoordinated contraction of ventricles can lead to EKG flatline

- Ventricular tachycardia: rate >120 beats/minute is an emergency situation in the case of prolonged duration with symptomatic patient.

V. Treatment

- Monitor cardiac activity.

- Early diagnosis and treatment are the cornerstones of therapy.

- In most cases, no treatment is needed.

- If the patient has low oxygen saturation levels, provide oxygen as needed.

- If complex abnormal beats are present with lack of blood flow to the heart or low blood pressure, use lidocaine to suppress PVCs.

- Correct electrolyte imbalances, particularly those of magnesium, calcium, and potassium.

- Acute lack of blood flow to the heart and/or heart attack may require airway intervention and cardiologist/advanced cardiovascular life support (ACLS) measures.

- Thrombolytic agents to remove blood clots

- Use of beta-blockade during the time following thrombolytic agent treatment when abnormal beats are frequently seen.

- Lidocaine is of benefit only with symptomatic, complex ectopy.

- Lidocaine is useful when symptomatic ectopy is associated with a longer-than-normal QT interval; it docs not lengthen the QT interval as other antiarrhythmic agents do.

- Give amiodarone to suppress ectopy/VT if it is significantly affecting blood flow. Additional beneficial effects include widening of coronary vessels and increased cardiac output.

Table 3.8 Pharmaceutical Treatment Options for PVCs

Drug Name	Class	Dosage	Considerations
Amiodarone (Cordarone)	Class III anti-arrhythmic	400 mg by mouth 3 times/day for 1 week; weekly reductions thereafter, with a goal of arriving at the lowest dose to get desired therapeutic benefit (usual maintenance dose is 200 mg/day)	During loading (initial, large dose in a series), patients must be monitored for slow heart arrhythmias. Before administration, control the ventricular rate and congestive heart failure (if present) with digoxin or calcium channel blockers.
Lidocaine (Dilocaine)	Class Ib anti-arrhythmic	1–1.5 mg/kg slow IV push over 2–3 minutes; may repeat dose of 0.5–0.75 mg/kg in 5–10 minutes up to 3 mg/kg total Continuous infusion 1–4 mg/minute Intramuscular (IM) injection: 300 mg (3 mg of 10% solution) in deltoid or hip.	IM dose indicated when IV administration is not possible or when EKG monitoring is not available and danger of ventricular arrhythmia is high
Procainamide (Procanbid)	Class Ia anti-arrhythmic	Capsules come in 250 mg; 375 mg; 500 mg. Controlled release tablets come in 500 mg; 750 mg; 1000 mg. *Intramuscular*: 0.5–1 g every 4–8 hours *Loading dose*: 100–200 mg/dose or 15–18 mg/kg; infuse slowly over 25–30 min; may repeat every 5 minutes as needed, not to exceed 1 g To convert from IV to oral, take total mg/hour IV dose, divide into 4 daily doses, and round to dosage form; immediate release should rarely be used.	IM: In patients with renal (kidney) impairment: reduce loading dose to 12 mg/kg. Maintenance: 1–4 mg/minute by continuous infusion Infusion: in patients with renal impairment: Reduce infusion to 1/3 in moderate renal or cardiac impairment and 2/3 in severe renal or cardiac impairment.

Drug Name	Class	Dosage	Considerations
Metoprolol (Lopressor)	Beta-adrenergic blocker Suppresses ventricular ectopy due to excess catecholamines	Tablets come in 25 mg; 50 mg; 100 mg; 200mg. *For acute tachyarrhythmias*: 5 mg IV over 1–2 minutes every 5–15 minutes; maximum 15 mg *For ventricular tachycardia* (off-label use): initial dose is 100 mg/day by mouth every day or divided 2–3 times/day; may increase every week as needed up to 450 mg/day	During IV administration, carefully monitor blood pressure, heart rate, and EKG.
Esmolol (Brevibloc)	Beta-adrenergic blocker Suppresses ventricular ectopy due to excess catecholamines	*For tachycardia/ hypertension*: Loading dose is 0.5 mg/kg IV over 1 minute, then Maintenance: start 0.05 mg/kg/minute IV for 4 minutes; may increase by 0.05 mg/kg up to 0.2 mg/kg/minute. If heart rate/blood pressure not controlled after 5 minutes, repeat bolus (500 mcg/kg/min for 1 minute), then start infusion of 100 mcg/kg/min IV. May administer a 3rd bolus if needed, then a maintenance infusion of 150 mcg/kg/min IV Higher maintenance doses may be required, up to 250–300 mcg/kg/min	Excellent drug for patients at risk of complications from beta-blockade, particularly those with reactive airway disease, mild-moderate left ventricular dysfunction, and/or peripheral vascular disease. Short half-life of 8 minutes allows titration to desired effect and quick discontinuation if necessary
Propranolol (Inderal)	Class II antiarrhythmic, nonselective beta-adrenergic receptor blocker with membrane-stabilizing activity that decreases automaticity of contractions	*Oral*: 10 mg by mouth every 6–8 hours; may increase dose every 3–7 days *IV*: 1–3 mg/dose IV at 1 mg/minute initially; repeat every 2–5 minutes to total of 5 mg. Once response or maximum dose is achieved, do not give additional dose for at least 4 hours.	Monitor blood pressure Less effective than thiazide diuretics in black and geriatric patients Shown to decrease mortality in hypertension and post-myocardial infarction

Drug Name	Class	Dosage	Considerations
Magnesium sulfate	Electrolyte Acts as antiarrhythmic agent, diminishes frequency of PVCs	With pulse (ACLS): 1–2 g slow IV (diluted in 50–100 mL 5% dextrose in water) over 5–60 minutes, then 0.5–1 g/hour IV infusion Cardiac arrest (ACLS): 1–2 g slow IV (diluted in 10 mL 5% dextrose in water) over 5–20 minutes	
Verapamil (Calan Covera Verelan)	Calcium depression of both impulse formation (automaticity) and conduction velocity	2.5–10 mg IV over 2 minutes May repeat 5–10 mg dose after 15–30 minutes or 0.075–0.15 mg/kg IV, up to 10 mg, over 2 minutes; may repeat once after 30 minutes Do not administer more than 10 mg/dose	Geriatric patients and those with liver impairment: lower dosage as recommended If renal impairment is present, monitor EKG.

###

References

Premature Ventricular Contractions. Mayo Clinic. www.mayoclinic.com/health/premature-ventricular-contractions/DS00949

Premature Ventricular Contractions. MedicineNet.com. www.medicinenet.com/premature_ventricular_contractions/page2.htm

Figure 3.21 Normal Sinus Rhythm. Source: Anthony Atkielski / Wikimedia Commons. Image at commons.wikimedia.org/wiki/File:SinusRhythmLabels.svg

Figure 3.22 Inverted T Wave in Lead V6. Source: Bron766, File:Tinvert (ECG).svg, CC-BY-SA-3.0. Image at commons.wikimedia.org/wiki/File:Tinvert_(ECG).svg

Ventricular Tachycardia
By Marian M. Houtman

Introduction

- Ventricular tachycardia (VT) is a heart rhythm that originates in the ventricles and produces a heart rate of at least 120 beats per minute (usually 150–200).

- Types of ventricular tachycardia:
    - **Non-sustained VT**: lasting less than 30 seconds
    - **Sustained VT**: lasting longer than 30 seconds

- Well-tolerated VT requires IV medications and monitoring.

- Symptomatic, hypotensive VT with a pulse requires synchronized cardioversion.

- Pulseless VT requires defibrillation and the same treatments as ventricular fibrillation (see "Ventricular Fibrillation" section in Chapter 3).

I. Basic Physiology

- Most common cause of VT is irritability of the ventricles
    - This can be caused by a lack of oxygen/blood to the heart muscle.

- Other causes include:
    - Electrolyte deficiencies: low potassium, low calcium, or low magnesium
    - Illicit drugs: methamphetamine or cocaine
    - Systemic diseases:
        - Sarcoidosis
        - Systemic lupus erythematous
        - Hemochromatosis
        - Rheumatoid arthritis
    - Congenital disorders, such as right ventricular dysplasia and tetralogy of Fallot
    - Prescribed drugs:
        - Digitalis toxicity
        - Those that prolong QT complex

- ▶ Type 1A antidysrhythmics
- ▶ Droperidol
- ▶ Related phenothiazines
- ○ Direct stimulation of the heart by improper central line placement
- ● VT must be strongly considered in any patient who faints and has the following risk factors:
  - ○ Prior heart attack(s)
  - ○ Structural heart disease
  - ○ Family history of premature sudden death
  - ○ Athletes: participation history and physical
  - ○ Family history of premature sudden cardiac death
  - ○ Evidence of cardiovascular disease
  - ○ Diseases of the heart muscle
  - ○ Ion channel disorders

II. Clinical Signs and Symptoms

- ● Pounding in the chest
- ● Lightheadedness
- ● Fainting: seen with heart structural damage
- ● Chest pain due to diminished blood flow to the heart may or may not be present.
- ● Ventricular tachycardia rhythm on monitor and 12-lead ECG
- ● Anxiety
- ● Sensation of neck fullness
- ● Shortness of breath

III. Diagnostic Work-up

- ● When VT is recognized, the rhythm should be quickly corrected.
- ● Defer much of the history and physical exam until the rhythm is corrected.
- ● Physical changes seen with VT:
  - ○ Cardiac output is reduced due to the fast heart rate and heart pump action.
  - ○ Congestive heart failure worsens.
  - ○ Hemodynamic (blood flow) collapse is likely.

○ If VT is tolerated, cardiomyopathy (weakening of heart muscle) will occur over a period of weeks to months, but resolves with successful management of VT.

● Perform a 12-lead ECG; factors that indicate presence of VT:

○ Rate >120 beats per minute (usually 150–200)

○ Wide QRS complexes (>140 mm; see Figure 3.23) in the same shape

○ Presence of atrioventricular (AV) dissociation (atria and ventricles with independent rhythms)

○ Fusion beats (when normal beat and ventricular beat coincide to make hybrid complex)

○ Capture beats (when SA node "captures" the ventricle)

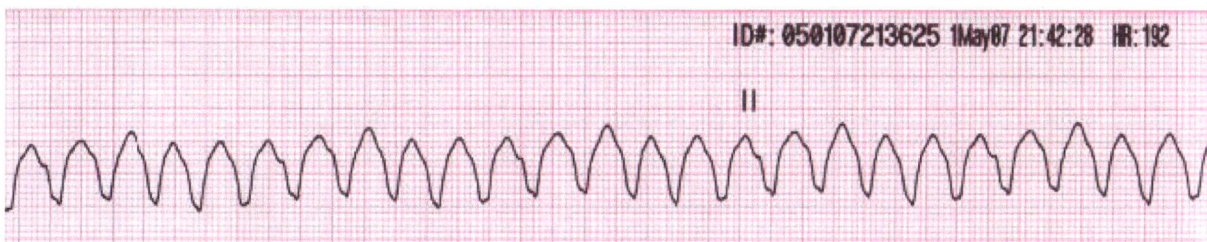

Figure 3.23 EKG Lead II: Ventricular Tachycardia.

● After rhythm is corrected, seek causes and treat to prevent recurrence.

○ Treat cardiovascular disease, conduction problems, etc., with medications or refer the patient for other therapies (e.g., ablation) as indicated.

○ If patient is <40 years old, evaluate for genetic arrhythmia syndromes, including:

▶ Long QT syndrome

▶ Short QT syndrome

▶ Right ventricular dysplasia

▶ Catecholamine-stimulated and hypertrophic cardiomyopathy

▶ Brugada syndrome

IV. Differential Diagnoses

● Atrial fibrillation

● Atrial flutter

● Atrial tachycardia

● Congestive heart failure and pulmonary edema

● Hypocalcemia (abnormally low level of calcium in the blood)

- Hypokalemia (abnormally low level of potassium in the blood)
- Hypomagnesemia (abnormally low level of magnesium in the blood)
- Myocardial infarction
- Paroxysmal supraventricular tachycardia
- Ventricular fibrillation

V. Treatment

- Treatments depend on how well the patient is tolerating VT. In general:
  - Well-tolerated VT requires IV medications and monitoring.
  - Symptomatic, hypotensive VT with a pulse requires synchronized cardioversion.
  - Pulseless VT requires defibrillation and the same treatments as ventricular fibrillation (see "Ventricular Fibrillation" section in Chapter 3).
- Interventions include:
  - Preparation of cardioversion equipment
  - Laboratory tests (when patient is stable)
    - Electrolyte levels: serum calcium, magnesium, and phosphate levels
    - Appropriate levels of therapeutic drugs (for example, digoxin). Toxicology screens may be helpful in those cases related to recreational drug use.
    - Evaluate for lack of blood flow to the heart or myocardial infarction, with serum cardiac troponin I or T levels or other cardiac markers
    - Potassium level: it is reasonable to maintain serum potassium levels above 4 mm/L in patients with acute myocardial infarction.
  - If patient becomes unstable (hypotensive), start advanced life support measures.
    - Provide cardioversion immediately at 100 joules (biphasic monitor).
    - Initiate airway interventions or CPR as necessary.
    - Establish vascular access.
    - Start amiodarone (in cardiac arrest situations, it is the drug of choice).
    - Initiate supplemental oxygen.
    - Monitor EKG rhythm strip.
    - If not in a medical support setting, transport the patient to one.
    - If untreated, the rhythm is likely to worsen to ventricular fibrillation, then death.
  - If patient is stable, get 12-lead EKG.

- ▶ In clinically stable ventricular tachycardia, initiate anti-dysrhythmic drugs. Options include procainamide, lidocaine (first-line in ischemic patient), amiodarone, and a handful of intravenous beta-adrenergic blocking agents (metoprolol, esmolol, propranolol).

- ▶ Class Ia sodium channel blockers

  - ▷ Procainamide (Pronestyl, Procanbid)

  - ▷ Quinidine sulfate (Quinidex Extentabs)

  - ▷ Disopyramide (Norpace)

  - ▷ Tocainide (Tonocard)

  - ▷ Propafenone (Rythmol)

- ▶ Class IV calcium channel blockers

  - ▷ Verapamil (Calan)

  - ▷ Diltiazem (Cardizem)

● Monitor for congestive heart failure symptoms:

  ○ Blood pressure changes

  ○ Respiratory difficulty

  ○ Lung sounds

  ○ Congestion

● Monitor EKG strip for changes to ventricular fibrillation.

● In stable patient with myocardial infarction and ischemia ruled out:

  ○ Adenosine may be given to rule out SVT with aberrancy.

  ○ Move on to amiodarone infusion (150 mg over 10 minutes, initially).

● If medical therapy is unsuccessful and patient is decompensating, provide synchronized cardioversion (100 joules biphasic or 50–200 joules monophasic).

  ○ Provide sedation if blood pressure will tolerate it.

● If runs of polymorphic VT (beat-to-beat variation in appearance) are observed punctuated by sinus rhythm with QT prolongation, then attempts should be made to correct torsades (see next section of this manual) with magnesium, isoproterenol, and/or pacing. Phenytoin and lidocaine may also help by shortening the QT interval in this setting, but procainamide is contraindicated because of its QT-prolonging effects.

● Correct hypokalemia and stop any medications associated with QT-interval prolongation.

Table 3.9 Pharmaceutical Treatment Options for Ventricular Tachycardia

Drug Name (Generic/ Trade)	Class	Dosage	Indication
Procainamide	Class Ia antiarrhythmic used for VT that is resistant to defibrillation and epinephrine. It is indicated for ventricular arrhythmia, such as sustained VT.	IV: 0.5–1 g every 4–8 hours; loading dose (initial, larger-than-normal dose given in a series) 100–200 mg dose or 15–18 mg/kg; infuse slowly over 25–30 minutes; may repeat every 5 minutes, as needed, up to 1g. Reduce dose for renal (kidney) impairment to 12 mg/kg. Reduce dose for cardiac impairment to 6 mg/kg; maintenance is 1–4 mg/kg continuous IV. To convert from IV to oral intake, divide total mg/24 hour IV dose into 4 daily SR doses, then round to dosage form; immediate release should rarely be used.	Life-threatening ventricular arrhythmia Off-label use: A-fib/flutter, paroxysmal AT Consideration: To ensure that the drug is well tolerated, patients should be monitored by automatic data collection/reporting and serial EKGs during 5–6 half-lives.
Lidocaine	A class Ib antiarrhythmic Although lidocaine may terminate VT successfully, it may increase overall mortality.	10% solution 100 mg/mL as 3mL auto injector (in the deltoid or thigh) Injectable solution: 10 mg/mL and 20mg/mL In cardiac arrhythmia, administer 1–1.5 mg/kg slow IV bolus over 2–3 minutes; may repeat doses of 0.5–0.75 mg/kg in 5–10 minutes, up to 3 mg/kg total. Continuous infusion: 1–4 mg/minute; if not possible, use intraosseous (injecting into bone marrow), route (per mouth), or down endotracheal tube (breathing tube). Monitor ECG.	Acute management of ventricular arrhythmia (cardiac surgery, acute MI) Off-label: children with premature ventricular beats during cardiac arrest Intramuscular dose is indicated when IV administration is not possible or when EKG monitoring is not available and danger of ventricular arrhythmia is high.

Drug Name (Generic/Trade)	Class	Dosage	Indication
Amiodarone	**Drug of choice in the treatment of unstable ventricular arrhythmias.** Pre-hospital studies currently suggest that amiodarone is safe and effective for use in out-of-hospital cardiac arrest.	Injectable solution comes in 50 mg/mL. Tablet comes in 100 mg and 200 mg.—*By mouth*: load 800–1600 mg; by mouth daily for 1–3 weeks until response; for load greater than 1000 mg/day divide into 2–3 doses/day. Maintenance: 200–600 mg every day. *IV:* 150 mg IV bolus (fast, large injection) in 10 minutes, THEN, 1 mg/minute IV for 6 hours, THEN, 0.5 mg/minute IV for 18 hours. Per ACLS guidelines, in pulseless V-Fib or VT, 300 mg IV in a single dose after dose of epinephrine, if no initial response to defibrillation; may repeat 150 mg IV every 5–10 minutes; rapid IV push if pulseless/no blood pressure; not to exceed 2.2 g/day	Unstable ventricular arrhythmias, VT related to blood circulation, resistant to other antiarrhythmic agents. Off-label: resistant sustained or paroxysmal A-fib, paroxysmal supraventricular tachycardia, atrial flutter Consideration: start elderly patients at lower dose
Sotalol (Betapace)	Class III antidysrhythmic, a potassium channel-blocking drug with a weak beta-blocker cffcct	Tablet comes in 80 mg, 120 mg, 160 mg, 240 mg. Injectable solution comes in 15 mg/mL. — *By mouth*: start 80 mg by mouth every 12 hours; increase as needed 120–160 mg every 12 hours (2–3 days between increments). *IV, substitute for sotalol by mouth:* 75 mg IV infused over 5 hours every 12 hours initially; adjust dose if needed every 3 days, not to exceed 150 mg IV every 12 hours.	Ventricular arrhythmias such as sustained ventricular tachycardia. Monitor QT interval Drug resistant, life-threatening ventricular arrhythmias (may require up to 480–640 mg/day)

Drug Name (Generic/ Trade)	Class	Dosage	Indication
Mexiletine (Mexitil)	Class Ib antidysrhythmic Generally well tolerated Occasionally used for VT, responding to IV lidocaine. Felt to be safer than Ic drugs.	Capsule comes in 150 mg, 200 mg, 250 mg. In ventricular arrhythmias (life-threatening), 200–300 mg dose by mouth, 3 times/day; may increase to 400 mg every 8 hours; no more than 1200 mg every day. Take with food or antacid; therapeutic range 0.5–2.0 mg/L	Life-threatening ventricular arrhythmias Off-label: prevention of ventricular arrhythmia in acute-phase MI (no change in mortality)
Metoprolol (Lopressor, Toprol XL)	A selective beta1-adrenergic receptor blocker.	Injectable solution comes in 1mg/ mL. Oral comes in 25 mg, 50 mg, 100 mg, 200 mg. *For acute MI, early treatment:* 2.5–5 mg rapid IV every 2–5 minutes, up to 15 mg over 10–15 minutes, THEN 15 minutes after last IV and receiving 15 mg IV; 50 mg by mouth every 6 hours for 48 hours, THEN 50–100 mg by mouth every 12 hours If full IV dose not tolerated: 25–50 mg by mouth every 6 hours after last IV *For acute tachyarrhythmias:* 5 mg IV over 1–2 minutes every 5–15 minutes; maximum 15 mg *For VT (off-label use):* initial dose is 100 mg/day by mouth every day or divided 2–3 times/day; may increase every week as needed up to 450 mg/ day	During IV administration, carefully monitor the patient's blood pressure, heart rate, and EKGs. Less effective than thiazide diuretics in black and geriatric patients Shown to decrease mortality in hypertension and post-myocardial infarction

Drug Name (Generic/ Trade)	Class	Dosage	Indication
Esmolol (Brevibloc)	Class II antiarrhythmic that selectively blocks beta1-receptors; little/no effect on beta2-receptor types.	Infusion bag comes in 2 g/100 mL, 2.5 g/250 mL. Injectable comes in 10 mg/mL. Postoperative/gradual control: load 0.5 mg/kg over 1 minute, THEN 0.05 mg/kg/minute IV for 4 minutes. If inadequate response in 5 minutes, 2nd loading dose of 0.5 mg/kg/minute for 1 minute, THEN 0.1 mg/kg/minute	Supraventricular tachycardia and atrial fibrillation/flutter. Less effective than thiazide diuretics in black and geriatric patients. Shown to decrease mortality in hypertension and post-MI Not necessary to supplement dose; not dialyzable
Flecainide (Tambocor)	Class Ic antiarrhythmic for life-threatening ventricular arrhythmia. Greatest effect on the His–Purkinje system The effects on AV nodal conduction time and intra-atrial conduction times, although present, are less pronounced than are the drug's effects on ventricular conduction speed.	Tablet comes in 50 mg, 100 mg, 150 mg. Initial dose 50–100 mg by mouth twice/day; start in clinic For sustained VT, no more than 400 mg/day. For paroxysmal supraventricular tachycardia, no more than 300 mg/day	Prevention of paroxysmal A-Fib/A-Flutter, paroxysmal supraventricular tachycardia, life-threatening ventricular arrhythmia In the presence of liver impairment: monitor plasma levels, reduce dose as necessary Administration: may take with food
Propafenone (Rythmol)	Used to treat life-threatening arrhythmias.	Tablet comes in 150 mg, 225 mg, 300 mg. Capsule comes in 225 mg, 325 mg, 425 mg. For ventricular arrhythmias, initial dose is 225 mg by mouth every 12 hours; may increase dose every 5 days to 325 mg by mouth every 12 hours, 425 mg by mouth every 12 hours if necessary	Life-threatening ventricular arrhythmias, paroxysmal A-Fib/A-Flutter, paroxysmal supraventricular tachycardia Off-label: A-Fib/A-Flutter with Wolff–Parkinson–White syndrome In patients with liver impairment, start with 20–30% of normal dose

Drug Name (Generic/Trade)	Class	Dosage	Indication
Quinidine (Quinidex, Quinora, Quinalan, Cardioquin)	Class Ia antiarrhythmic Indicated for VT	Tablet (controlled-release) comes in 300 mg, 324 mg. Tablet comes in 200 mg, 300 mg. Syrup comes in 10 mg/mL. Injectable comes in 80 mg/mL. *Test dose*: 200 mg by mouth quinidine sulfate several hours before full dosage is administered *For atrial/ventricular premature contractions*: 200–300 mg by mouth 3–4 times/day; maintenance is 200–400 mg by mouth 3–4 times/day or 600 mg of SR (controlled release) by mouth every 8–12 hours; do not administer more than 3–4 grams per day	Cardioversion or chronic therapy for A-fib/flutter, paroxysmal supraventricular tachycardia, malaria Off-label: prevention of atrial, AV junctional, and ventricular premature complexes in adults; paroxysmal atrial tachycardia or AV junctional rhythm, paroxysmal VT, pseudobulbar affect (condition in which one suddenly starts to laugh or cry)

###

VI. Prognosis

- Patient's left ventricular function is the best predictor.
- Patients with non-sustained VT and ischemic cardiomyopathy have a sudden cardiac death incidence of 30% within 2 years.
- Patients with VT and no heart disease have an excellent prognosis unless mortally injured due to injuries sustained during fainting spells (e.g., falls, drowning).
- Patients with QT syndrome, right ventricular dysplasia, and hypertrophic cardiomyopathy may be at increased risk of sudden death.

References

Heart and Blood Disorders. Merck Manuals.
www.merckmanuals.com/professional/cardiovascular-disorders/arrhythmias-and-conduction-disorders/ventricular-tachycardia

Figure 3.23 EKG Lead II: Ventricular Tachycardia. Source: Glenlarson / Wikimedia Commons / Public Domain. Image at
en.wikipedia.org/wiki/File:Lead_II_rhythm_ventricular_tachycardia_Vtach_VT.JPG

Torsades de Pointes

By Marian M. Houtman

Introduction

- Torsades de pointes is an uncommon form of ventricular tachycardia (VT).
  - Often referred to as polymorphic ventricular tachycardia
- It is characterized by a gradual change in amplitude (height) and twisting of the QRS complexes around an imaginary middle/zero line.
- This is a life-threatening arrhythmia.
- Has prolonged QT interval (usually 600 msec or more)
- May be congenital (present at birth) or acquired
- Stops spontaneously, but may return and lead to ventricular fibrillation (V-fib)
- Ventricular rate can range from 150 to 250 beats per minute.
- Presence is an indication for magnesium administration.

I. Pathophysiology

- Associated with prolonged (longer than normal) QT intervals
- Congenital long QT syndrome (Jervell and Lange–Nielsen; Romano–Ward syndromes)
- Acquired long QT; antiarrhythmic drugs associated with torsades include the following:
  - Class IA: quinidine, disopyramide, procainamide
  - Class III: sotalol, amiodarone (rare), ibutilide, dofetilide, almokalant
  - Class IC: encainide, flecainide
- Other drug classes associated with torsades include the following:
  - Antibiotics: erythromycin, clarithromycin, azithromycin, levofloxacin, moxifloxacin, gatifloxacin, trimethoprim/sulfa-methoxazole, clindamycin, pentamidine, chloroquine
  - Antifungals: ketoconazole, itraconazole
  - Antivirals: amantadine
  - Antipsychotics: haloperidol, phenothiazines, thioridazine, trifluoperazine, sertindole, zimeldine, ziprasidone
  - Tricyclic or tetracyclic antidepressants

- ○ Lithium

- ○ Antihistamines (histamine1-receptor antagonists): terfenadine (no longer sold in US), astemizole (no longer sold in US), diphenhydramine, hydroxyzine:

  - ▶ Astemizole, terfenadine, in high dosages or if used in combination with azole anti-fungal drugs or macrolide antibiotics, may cause torsades, sudden death.

  - ▶ Grapefruit juice may slow the liver's metabolism of these antihistamines, and prolong the QT interval in patients taking astemizole or terfenadine.

- ○ Cholinergic antagonists: cisapride, organophosphates (pesticides)

- ○ Diuretics: indapamide, hydrochlorothiazide, furosemide

- ○ Antihypertensives: bepridil (no longer sold in the United States), lidoflazine, prenyl-amine, ketanserin

- ○ Anthracycline chemotherapeutic agents (doxorubicin, daunomycin)

- ○ Anticonvulsants: phenytoin, carbamazepine

- ○ Highly active antiretroviral drugs

- ○ High-dose methadone

- ○ Cocaine

- ○ Some fluoroquinolones (and any other medication using the CYP3A metabolic pathway)

- ○ Oral hypoglycemics

- ○ Citrate, the anticoagulant used in blood products, when massive blood transfusion is given

- ○ Vasopressin (possible)

- ○ Fluoxetine (possible)

- ○ Ranolazine, an antiangina agent, prolongs QT interval, but torsades is rare.

- ● Conditions associated with torsades:

  - ○ Electrolyte abnormalities: low potassium, low magnesium, low calcium levels

  - ○ Endocrine disorders: hypothyroidism, hyperparathyroidism, pheochromocytoma, hyperaldosteronism

  - ○ Cardiac conditions: myocardial ischemia, myocardial infarction, myocarditis, bradyar-rhythmia, complete atrioventricular block, takotsubo cardiomyopathy

  - ○ Intracranial disorders: subarachnoid hemorrhage, thalamic hematoma, cerebrovascular accident, encephalitis, head injury

  - ○ Nutritional disorders: anorexia nervosa, starvation, liquid protein diets, gastroplasty and ileojejunal bypass, celiac disease

- Other risk factors: female sex, white individuals, baseline cardiographic abnormalities, kidney or liver failure

II. Clinical Signs and Symptoms

- History of repeated, unprovoked heart pounding episodes with associated dizziness, fainting, nausea, cold sweats, shortness of breath, chest pain.
- Sudden cardiac death (may be the first event)
- Family history of sudden cardiac death
- Prolonged QT interval
- A family history of congenital deafness; no QT prolongation.
- History of Romano–Ward syndrome (inherited disorder that causes long QT syndrome)
- Physical exam
  - Findings depend on the rate and duration of tachycardia and the degree of insufficient blood supply to the brain
  - May include: rapid pulse, low or normal BP, brief or prolonged loss of consciousness
  - May be preceded by a slow heart beat (bradycardia) or premature ventricular contractions (leading palpitations)
  - Pale color and excessive sweating may be noted, especially with a sustained episode.

III. Diagnostic Work-up

- EKG; frequent EKG monitoring for patients at risk
  - Examine patients in sinus rhythm; examine the QT interval if prolonged QT and pathological U waves present
  - Torsades-looking rhythm of 5–20 beats at a rate >200 beats/minute; sustained episodes occasionally can be seen
  - Twisting QRS complexes around imaginary zero line
    - ▶ Complete 180° twist (flip) of QRS complexes in 10–12 beats
  - First beat: short, followed by a full pause. Second beat: long, a longer QT interval. If the next beat follows soon after, this third beat will likely fall within the QT interval, resulting in an R-on-T.
    - ▶ May stop spontaneously, or change to a non-polymorphic VT or V-fib
  - T-wave alternans (variation in shape, height of T waves) may be seen before torsades.

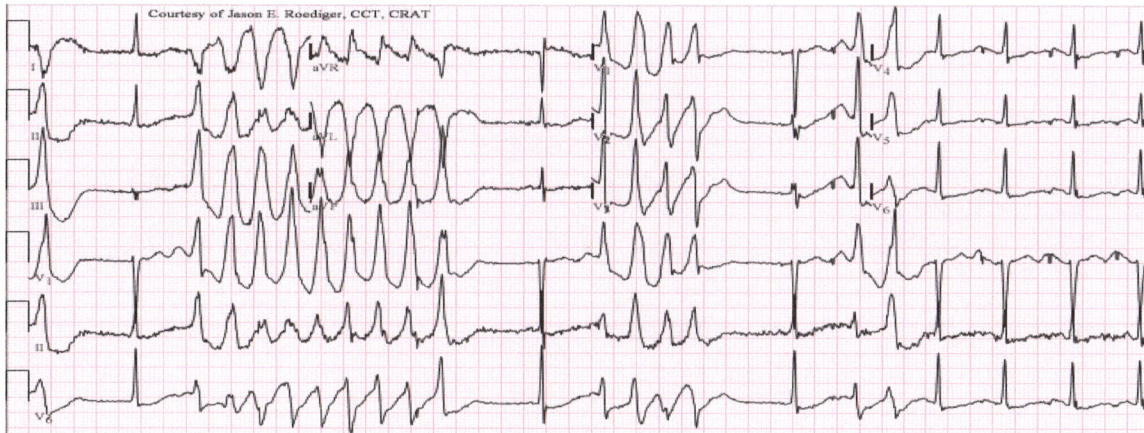

Figure 3.24 EKG of Torsades de Pointes.

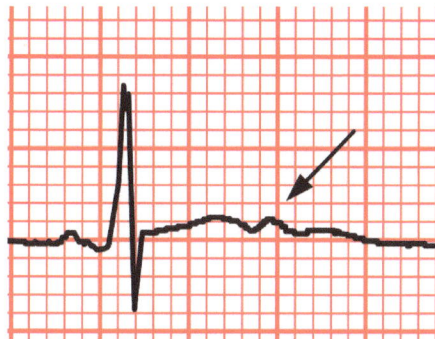

Figure 3.25 EKG A U Wave Most Often Seen in Hypokalemia; Also Seen in Hypercalcemia, Thyrotoxicosis, and Congenital Long QT Syndrome.

- Laboratory studies
  - Electrolytes: check for hypokalemia, hypomagnesemia, and hypocalcemia.
  - Cardiac enzymes
  - Rule out myocardial ischemia, especially in patients without QT prolongation.
- Imaging studies to rule out structural heart disease, if any clinical suggestion is present.
  - Chest radiographs
  - Echocardiography

IV. Differential Diagnoses

- Monomorphic ventricular tachycardia (QRS complexes look the same)
- Pediatrics tachycardia

- Fainting
- Chronic kidney failure and dialysis complication
- Toxicity, antidysrhythmics
- Toxicity, antihistamines
- Ventricular fibrillation
- Sudden cardiac death
- Supraventricular tachycardia with aberrant conduction (atrial fibrillation will be mixed with narrow typical QRS complexes)

V. Treatment

- **Short-term:**
  - Beta 1–adrenergic stimulation (in *acquired* torsades patients only)
  - Remove/correct any causes of torsades
  - Treat any predisposing condition (electrolyte abnormalities, bradycardia)
  - Magnesium is the drug of choice.
    - ▶ Can be given at 1–2 g IV initially in 30–60 seconds, which can be repeated in 5–15 minutes
    - ▶ *OR* a continuous infusion can be started at a rate of 3–10 mg/minutes.
  - Magnesium is effective even in patients with normal levels. Because of the danger of hypomagnesemia (depression of neuromuscular function), closely monitor patient.
  - Supplemental potassium to increase concentration to high normal level.
  - Isoproterenol can be used in bradycardia-dependent torsades that is usually associated with acquired long QT syndrome (pause-dependent).
    - ▶ Administered as a continuous IV infusion to keep the heart rate above 90 beats per minute.
    - ▶ Contraindicated in congenital form of long QT syndrome.
    - ▶ It is used as interim agent until overdrive pacing can be started.
  - Temporary transvenous pacing
    - ▶ Pacing is effective in both forms of the long QT syndrome because it facilitates the repolarizing potassium currents and prevents long pauses.
    - ▶ Atrial pacing is the preferred mode because it preserves the atrial contribution to ventricular filling and also results in a narrower QRS complexes and shorter QT.
    - ▶ In patients with AV block, ventricular pacing can be used to suppress torsades.

- ▶ Pacing should begin at a rate of 90–110 bpm until the QT interval is normalized.
- ▶ Overdrive pacing may be necessary at a rate of up to 140 bpm to control the rhythm.
- ○ If patient deteriorates to ventricular fibrillation, defibrillation should be performed.
- **Long-term:**
  - ○ Mexiletine may be helpful in suppressing torsades.
  - ○ If torsades returns, try a short-acting beta-blocker (e.g., esmolol).
  - ○ Congenital long QT
    - ▶ Propranolol, esmolol or nadolol are beta-adrenergic antagonists, used as a first-line, long-term therapy in congenital long QT syndrome at maximal doses.
    - ▶ Avoid beta-blockers in congenital cases in which bradycardia is a prominent feature.
    - ▶ Competitive sports is prohibited in patients with congenital long QT syndrome.
  - ○ Beta blockers are contraindicated in acquired long QT syndrome.
  - ○ Permanent pacing, if patient continues to have symptoms after receiving the maximally tolerated dose of beta-blockers. Pacing can be used in combination with beta blockers.
  - ○ Implantable cardioverter-defibrillators (ICDs), if torsades returns despite treatment with beta blockers and pacing; beta-blockers should be used along with ICDs.
  - ○ Patients without fainting, ventricular tachyarrhythmia, or a family history of sudden cardiac death can be observed without starting any treatment.
  - ○ Acquired long QT
    - ▶ Long-term treatment is usually not required because the QT interval returns to normal after underlying factors or predisposing conditions are corrected.
    - ▶ Pacemaker implantation is effective in cases associated with heart block or bradycardia. ICDs can be used for torsades not corrected by avoidance of the underlying factors.
  - ○ The boundary between acquired and congenital torsades may not always be clear. Additional factors are often present, and individuals may show increased susceptibility to QT effects.
    - ▶ Refer patient for consultation with cardiologist, hospitalization.

Table 3.10 Pharmaceutical Treatment Options for Torsades de Pointes

Drug Name (Generic/ Trade)	Class	Dosage	Consideration
Esmolol (Brevibloc)	Beta-adrenergic blocker Suppresses ventricular ectopy due to excess catecholamines.	*For tachycardia/ hypertension, load*: 0.5 mg/kg IV over 1 minute, THEN initiate maintenance; start 0.05 mg/kg/minute IV for 4 minutes; may increase by 0.05 mg/kg up to 0.2 mg/kg/minute If heart rate/blood pressure not controlled after 5 minutes, repeat bolus (500 mcg/kg/minute for 1 minute), then initiate infusion of 100 mcg/kg/minute IV May administer a 3rd bolus if needed, followed by a maintenance infusion of 150 mcg/kg/min IV Higher maintenance doses may be required, up to 250–300 mcg/kg/minute	Excellent drug for patients at risk of complications from beta-blockade, particularly those with reactive airway disease, mild-moderate left ventricular dysfunction, and/or peripheral vascular disease. Short half-life of 8 minutes allows titration to desired effect and quick discontinuation if necessary
Propranolol (Inderal)	Class II anti-arrhythmic, nonselective beta-adrenergic receptor blocker with membrane-stabilizing activity that decreases automaticity of contractions.	*Orally*: 10 mg by mouth every 6–8 hours; may increase dose every 3–7 days *IV*: 1–3 mg/dose IV at 1 mg/minute initially; repeat every 2–5 minutes to total of 5mg Once response or maximum dose achieved, do not give additional dose for at least 4 hours	Monitor blood pressure Less effective than thiazide diuretics in black and geriatric patients Shown to decrease mortality in hypertension and post-myocardial infarction
Magnesium sulfate	Electrolyte. Acts as antiarrhythmic agent, diminishes frequency of PVCs	In patients with detectable pulse (per ACLS guidelines), starting dose is 1–2 g slow IV (diluted in 50–100 mL 5% dextrose in water) over 5–60 minutes, THEN 0.5–1 g/hour IV infusion In cardiac arrest (per ACLS guidelines), administer 1–2 g slow IV (diluted in 10 mL % dextrose in water) over 5–20 minutes	

Drug Name (Generic/ Trade)	Class	Dosage	Consideration
Isoproterenol (Isuprel)	Acts exclusively on beta receptors	Start at lowest possible dose. *IV injection:* Dilute 1 mL (0.02 mg) to 10 mL with sodium chloride injection or 5% dextrose injection Initial dose: 0.02 mg to 0.06 mg 1 mL to 3 mL of diluted solution. Repeat doses: 0.01 mg to 0.2 mg (0.5 mL to 10 mL diluted solution) IV solution: dilute 10 mL (2 mg) in 500 mL 5% dextrose solution 5 mcg/minute or 1.23 mL diluted solution per minute	Do not use with epinephrine

VI. Complications and Prognosis

- Monomorphic ventricular tachycardia
- Ventricular fibrillation
- Sudden cardiac death
- In patients with congenital long QT syndrome, mortality rate for untreated patients is 50% in 10 years, which can be reduced to 3–4% with therapeutic intervention.
- In patients with acquired long QT syndrome, prognosis is excellent once the underlying factor has been identified and reliably withheld.

VII. Patient Education

- Instruct patients to use medications only with the approval of a physician or medic.
- Instruct patients to avoid competitive sports (in cases of congenital long QT syndrome).
- Teach patients how to monitor pulse and recognize adverse drug effects.
- Families should undergo training for basic life support.

References

Dave, Jatin. Torsade de Pointes. Medscape. emedicine.medscape.com/article/1950863-overview

Figure 3.24 EKG of Torsades de Pointes. Source: Jer5150 / Wikimedia Commons / CC-BY-SA-3.0. Image at commons.wikimedia.org/wiki/File:Torsades_de_Pointes_TdP.png

Figure 3.25 EKG A U Wave Most Often Seen in Hypokalemia; Also Seen in Hypercalcemia, Thyrotoxicosis, and Congenital Long QT Syndrome. Source: James Heilman, MD / Wikimedia Commons / CC-BY-SA-3.0. Image at commons.wikimedia.org/wiki/File:U_wave.svg

Ventricular Fibrillation
By Marian M. Houtman

Introduction

- Ventricular fibrillation (V-fib or VF) is the uncoordinated contraction of the ventricular heart muscle; it quivers rather than contracts.

- VF is the most commonly identified arrhythmia in cardiac-arrest patients.

- Pulses are absent at major pulse points (carotid or femoral arteries).

- VF is a medical emergency that requires prompt basic life support.

- If VF continues for more than a few seconds, the patient's chances for survival diminish.

I. Pathophysiology

- VF is most often caused by a sudden lack of blood to the heart from a heart attack due to coronary artery disease.

- Risk factors for VF that involve structural heart disease include:

  ○ Heart disease

  ○ Congenital heart disease

  ○ Cardiomyopathy: conditions in which the heart muscle weakens, enlarges, or thickens are the second most important cardiac causes of sudden death.

  ○ Aortic stenosis: aortic valve narrows

  ○ Aortic dissection: separation of the layers forming the aortic wall

  ○ Pericardial tamponade: fluid build-up between the heart and pericardial sac

  ○ Myocarditis: inflammation of the myocardium

- Risk factors for VF that are cardiac in origin, but do not involve structural heart disease, include:

  ○ Catecholaminergic polymorphic ventricular tachycardia: in genetically predisposed individuals, usually occurs during exercise and causes fainting.

  ○ Tachycardia originating in the outflow tract of the right ventricle

  ○ Electrical activity disruption after blunt trauma to the heart (e.g., being struck)

  ○ Ventricles that contract too early, possibly due to an extra, abnormal pathway (including Wolff–Parkinson–White syndrome)

- Heart block
- QT interval that is abnormally long, often due to medication, showing upward then downward pointing QRS complexes, with a twisted appearance (torsades de pointes)
- Disorders of ion channels: long QT, short QT syndromes, or Brugada syndrome
- Risk factors for VF that are respiratory in origin include lack of oxygen from:
  - Bronchial spasm
  - Aspiration (inhalation of a foreign substance)
  - Drowning
  - Sleep apnea
  - Pulmonary embolism
  - Tension pneumothorax (presence of air in the space surrounding the lung[s])
- Metabolic or toxic risk factors include:
  - Electrolyte disturbances and acidosis
  - Medications or drug ingestion
  - Environmental poisoning
  - Sepsis: the body's attempt to fight infection causes inflammation throughout the body
- Neurologic risk factors include:
  - Seizure
  - Cerebrovascular accident (stroke)

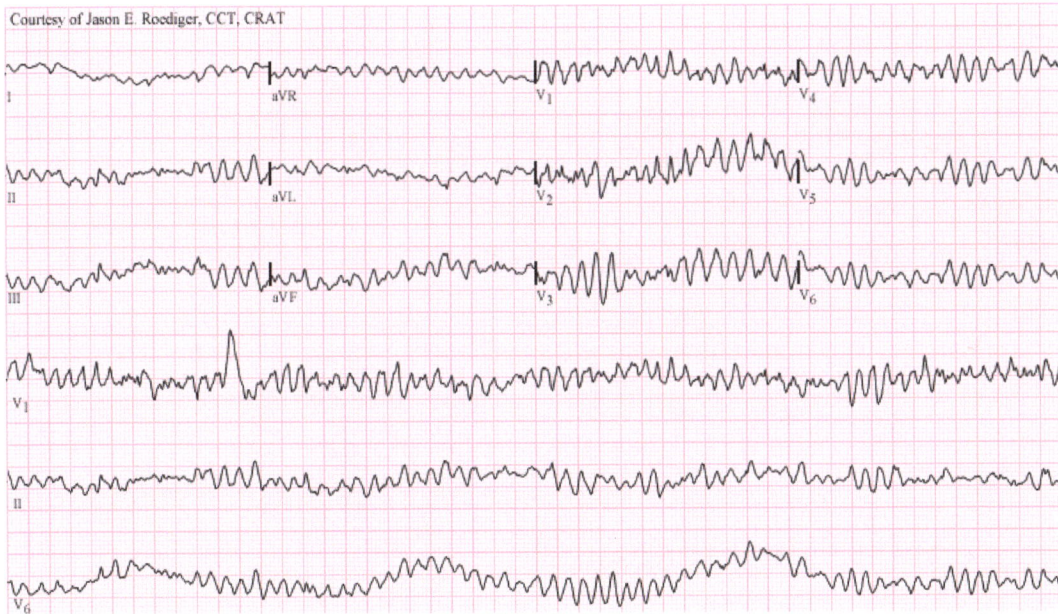

Figure 3.26 EKG Showing Ventricular Fibrillation. No clear QRS complex is seen and electrical activity is disorganized. It is *not* appropriate to obtain a 12-lead ECG of VF when it is recognized on the monitor in a pulseless patient. Priorities include CPR and ACLS interventions.

II. Clinical Signs and Symptoms

- Ventricular fibrillation often occurs without warning.

- Short-lived symptoms can include:

  - Chest pain

  - Shortness of breath

  - Pounding in chest

  - Fainting

  - Increase in heart rate

  - Premature ventricular contractions (PVCs)

  - Period of ventricular tachycardia

- Patients with VF will lose consciousness and have no pulse or respirations.

  - Take no more than 10 seconds to check for a pulse.

  - May have ineffective, agonal breaths (dying gasps)

  - If no pulse is found, proceed with chest compressions.

- Initiate cardiopulmonary resuscitation (CPR).

- Monitor will show VF, which requires defibrillation as soon as it is available.

III. Diagnostic Work-up

- The VF patient requires immediate CPR and prompt defibrillation to recover a perfusing rhythm.

  ○ Perform advanced cardiovascular life support (ACLS) assessment and interventions and defer other diagnostics of no immediate benefit.

  ○ All lab tests, ECGs, and imaging are deferred until return of spontaneous circulation is assured.

  ○ Tests will be targeted toward the suspected cause of the arrest.

IV. Differential Diagnoses

- Hyperkalemia
- Hypokalemia
- Torsade de Pointes
- Antidepressant toxicity
- Cocaine toxicity
- Digitalis toxicity
- Ventricular tachycardia

V. Treatment

- Because of the critical importance of early defibrillation, pre-hospital care is vital for arrests due to ventricular fibrillation (VF) that occur outside the hospital. Bystander CPR slows the degeneration of VF and improves survival. Automated external defibrillators (AEDs) are easily used by lay providers and in some countries are available in many public areas.

- ACLS algorithm for VF

  ○ Health care providers should have adequate training and equipment to manage cardiac arrest; American Heart Association ACLS guidelines are updated every 5 years and will supersede any material that becomes dated here.

  ○ Immediately initiate CPR and give oxygen by bag-valve-mask when available.

  ○ Apply monitor and verify patient is in VF as soon as possible.

  ○ Defibrillate once.

    ▶ **Adults:** device-specific or 150 joules for biphasic waveform and 360 joules for monophasic waveform

- ▶ **Children**: 2 J/kg
- ○ Resume CPR immediately without pulse check and continue for 5 cycles.
- ○ One cycle of CPR equals 30 compressions and 2 breaths.
- ○ Five cycles of CPR should take roughly 2 minutes (compression rate 100 per minute).
- ○ Do not check for rhythm/pulse until 5 cycles of CPR are completed.
- ○ During CPR, minimize interruptions while the following are performed:
  - ▶ Secure intravenous access.
  - ▶ If advanced airway is placed, continue CPR at 100 compressions per minute without pauses for respirations, and administer respirations at 8–10 breaths per minute (one breath every 6–8 seconds).
- ○ Check rhythm after 2 minutes of CPR.
- ○ Repeat a single defibrillation if still in VF or pulseless VT with rhythm check. Can use escalating doses. For children, use 4 J/kg for second and all subsequent defibrillations.
- ○ Resume CPR for 2 minutes immediately after defibrillation.
- ○ Continuously repeat the cycle of the following:
  - ▶ Rhythm check
  - ▶ Defibrillation
  - ▶ 2 minutes of CPR
- ○ Vasopressors
  - ▶ Give vasopressor during CPR before or after shock when intravenous or intraosseous (IO) access (into the bone marrow) is available.
  - ▶ Administer epinephrine 1 mg every 3–5 minutes, beginning after the second defibrillation.
  - ▶ Consider giving vasopressin 40 units to replace either the first or second epinephrine dose.
- ○ Antidysrhythmics
  - ▶ Give antidysrhythmic during CPR before or after shock.
  - ▶ Administer amiodarone 300 mg IV/IO once after the third defibrillation, then consider administering an additional 150 mg once.
  - ▶ As an alternative to amiodarone, administer lidocaine 1–1.5 mg/kg first dose, then additional 0.5 mg/kg doses up to a maximum total of 3 mg/kg.
  - ▶ If rhythm is suggestive of torsades de pointes, administer 1–2 g magnesium IV/IO.
  - ▶ Administer sodium bicarbonate 1 mEq/kg IV/IO in cases of known or suspected pre-existent hyperkalemia or tricyclic antidepressant overdose.

▶ Lidocaine and epinephrine can be administered through the endotracheal (ET) tube if IV/IO attempts fail. Use 2.5 times the IV dose.

○ Correct the following if necessary and/or possible:

▶ Hypovolemia (low blood volume): provide isotonic crystalloid and blood products, if indicated.

▶ Hypoxia (lacking oxygen): improve airway/oxygenation

▶ Hydrogen ion (acidosis): improve airway/oxygenation and consider bicarbonate therapy.

▶ Hyper/hypokalemia (too much or too little potassium) and metabolic disorders

▶ Hypoglycemia (low blood sugar): check fingerstick or administer glucose

▶ Hypothermia: check core rectal temperature

▶ Toxins: seek family member or friend who can provide history of ingestion/exposure.

▶ Cardiac tamponade: check via ultrasonography and consider pericardiocentesis (procedure that uses a needle to remove fluid from the pericardial sac [the tissue that surrounds the heart]).

▶ Tension pneumothorax: perform immediate needle thoracostomy (procedure used to remove air from around the lungs) and follow-up with chest tube.

▶ Blood clots, coronary or pulmonary: consider thrombolytic therapy if suspected, and in the case of MI, arrange for heart catheterization lab **immediately** if return of spontaneous circulation (ROSC) and stabilization are achieved.

▶ Trauma: stop the bleeding, provide IV fluids, blood products, and arrange for surgery **immediately** if ROSC achieved.

○ Refractory or recurrent VF

▶ Lack of response to standard defibrillation algorithms is challenging.

▶ If ongoing lack of blood supply is the suspected cause of recurrent VF, consider emergent cardiac catheterization and angioplasty (procedure to open blocked or narrow arteries), and intra-aortic balloon pump placement.

○ Post-resuscitative care

▶ Antidysrhythmics used successfully should be continued.

▷ After initial amiodarone bolus of 150 mg over 10 minutes, consider continued amiodarone therapy with 1 mg/minute IV for 6 hours, then 0.5 mg/minute for 18 hours.

▷ Or lidocaine at 1–4 mg/minute

▶ Support low blood pressure by administering 1–2 liters crystalloid and a vasopressor infusion like dopamine or norepinephrine as needed.

- ▶ Check for complications (e.g., aspiration pneumonia, CPR-related injuries).

- ▶ Determine need for emergent interventions (thrombolytics, antidotes, decontamination).

- ▶ "Cardiocerebral resuscitation" approach; the 3 pillars of this approach are as follows:

  - ▷ Cardiopulmonary resuscitation without mouth-to-mouth ventilations or continuous chest compressions (CCC) for all patients with witnessed cardiac arrest.

  - ▷ Give 200 CCC before and after a single defibrillation for patients with arrest lasting longer than 5 minutes (circulatory phase of arrest). Repeat 3 times before endotracheal intubation. Epinephrine should be given as soon as IV or intraosseous access available.

  - ▷ Post-resuscitation care may include mild cooling (hypothermia) of patients in coma, and urgent cardiac catheterization including percutaneous coronary intervention as needed, unless otherwise contraindicated by trauma, instability, or other criteria.

VI. Mortality/Morbidity

- ● Patients who have a witnessed cardiac arrest have improved outcomes, especially those patients with an initial rhythm of ventricular fibrillation who receive bystander CPR, and receive defibrillation and advanced cardiac life support from emergency medical services personnel within 10 minutes of onset.

- ● Black males have the highest incidence of sudden cardiac death.

References

Intraosseous Infusion. Wikipedia. en.wikipedia.org/wiki/Intraosseous_infusion

Jatin, Dave. Ventricular Fibrillation in Emergency Medicine. Medscape. emedicine.medscape.com/article/760832-overview

Figure 3.26 EKG Showing Ventricular Fibrillation. Source: Jer5150 / Wikimedia Commons / CC-BY-SA-3.0 / GNU Free Documentation License. Image at en.wikipedia.org/wiki/File:Ventricular_fibrillation.png

Chapter 4:

Venous Disease

Varicose Veins
By Marian M. Houtman

Introduction

- Varicose veins are twisted, enlarged veins most commonly found in the legs and feet.

- This condition can occur when veins cannot carry blood back to the heart (venous insufficiency), causing long-term pressure on the weakened veins of the lower body.

- Symptoms may be mild with the patient complaining of discomfort while standing, or cosmetically disfiguring. Over time, the patient may complain of serious pain, and as the condition becomes more severe, loss of limb may result.

- Spider veins are a mild, common form of varicose veins.

I. Pathophysiology

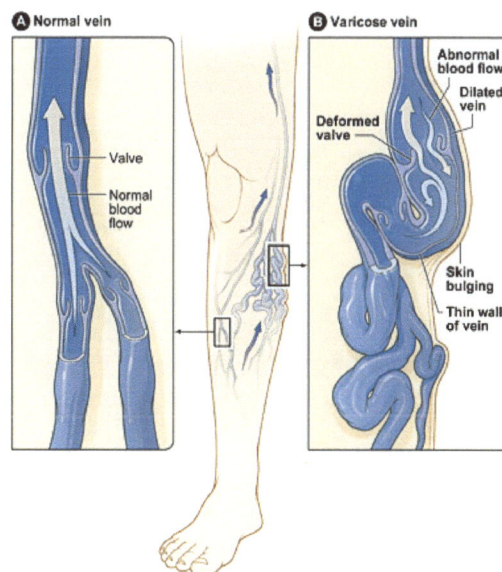

Figure 4.1 Normal and Varicose Veins. (A) The normal vein shows one-way flow of blood in a nondilated vein. (B) Varicose vein shows the convoluted, enlarged vein with a weakened valve; blood flows in different directions, causing the bulging vein effect you see on inspection of the leg skin surface.

II. Clinical Signs and Symptoms

- Spider veins (small dilated blood vessels near the surface of the skin)
- Burning sensations
- Swelling of leg (edema)
- Throbbing
- Cramping and leg fatigue
- Complaints decrease with walking or elevation.
- Leg heaviness, throbbing, dull ache that becomes worse when standing for long periods of time
- Discomfort with extended standing exercise
- Pain or tenderness along the course of a vein
- Pruritus (itching)
- Restless legs
- Night cramps, muscle fatigue
- Skin changes
- Numbness of legs, feet (paresthesias)
- Open sores (ulceration)

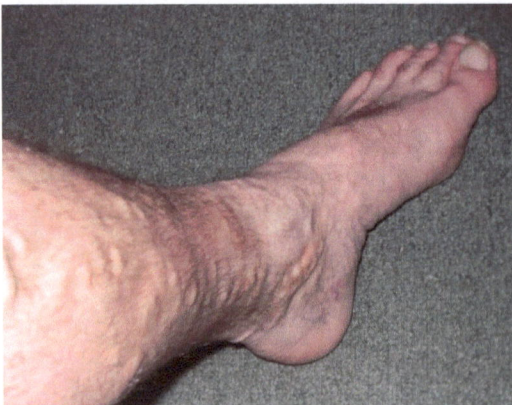

Figure 4.2 Skin Changes Commonly Seen in Varicose Veins.

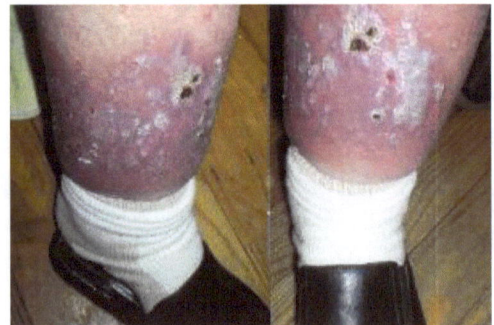

Figure 4.3 Leg Ulcers.

Table 4.1 Characteristics of Varicose Veins

	Appearance	Symptoms	Causes
Spider Veins	A web-like network of veins, appearing near the surface of skin of legs or feet; may be red or blue in color. Cosmetic concern.	Painless, or itching, burning sensation with prolonged standing.	Increasing age, pregnancy (hormones). Risk factors: age, female gender, heredity, obesity, standing or sitting for long periods of time
Varicose Veins	Winding, enlarged, twisted, bulging dilated veins found in legs and feet.	Dark purple, blue in color Pain, soreness, burning, aching, heavy feeling, throbbing, cramping May have cellulitis or ulceration, present history of hemorrhage (escape of blood from a ruptured blood vessel) or thrombophlebitis (vein inflammation related to a blood clot).	Increasing age, pregnancy (hormones). Risk factors: age, female gender, heredity, obesity, standing or sitting for long periods of time

III. Diagnostic Work-up

- Assess for varicose veins by having the patient stand.
  - Inspect from front of thighs to side of legs (long saphenous veins)
  - Inspect back of calves (short saphenous vein)
  - Look for dilated, twisted veins, and determine site of valve that is not properly performing.
- Examine skin for:
  - Eczema (scaly, itchy redness, oozing or crusting)
  - Brown discoloration of leg
  - Thin skin
  - Ulcers, especially on the bony areas on the outside of the ankles
  - Tenderness (inflammation, swelling)

○ Hardness (blood clot)

○ Thick, hard skin

○ Scarred, white patches

● Perform cough impulse test

○ Patient stands and holds fingers over saphenofemoral opening (see Figure 4.4).

○ Patient coughs; if saphenofemoral valve is not closing properly, cough makes a fluid "buzzing feeling" or thrill (a vibration felt on palpation).

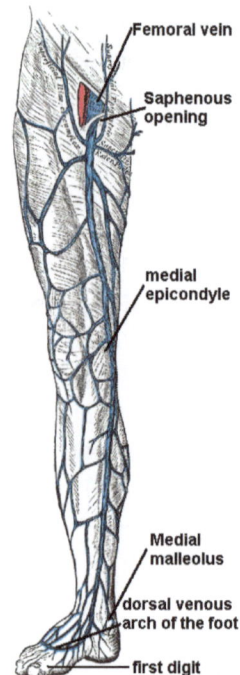

Figure 4.4 The Saphenofemoral Opening. Located 5 cm below and medial to the femoral pulse.

● Perform Trendelenberg test

○ Purpose: To find how far up the leg the improperly functioning valves are located.

○ Patient lies flat, leg is elevated.

○ Tie tourniquet around thigh at saphenous opening.

▶ Use 2 fingers if no tourniquet is available.

○ Patient stands.

○ If the valve at the tourniquet site is normal, blood will slowly fill the vein from below the tourniquet.

○ If the valve is incompetent, a sudden gush will fill the vein from above when tourniquet is removed.

- ○ The procedure can be repeated down the leg until the improperly functioning valve is found.
- ● Perthes's test
  - ○ Similar to Trendelenburg test
  - ○ Release a bit of the tourniquet, then have the patient rise up and down on toes.
  - ○ If the calf veins have properly functioning valves, the varicose veins will become less tense.
- ● Ultrasound
  - ○ Look for evidence of blood clots
  - ○ Rule out deep vein thrombosis (DVT), the formation of a blood clot in a deep vein in the leg.
  - ○ This is a non-invasive test.
  - ○ With information on local valve function, an anatomic map of disease may be constructed.

IV. Differential Diagnosis

- ● DVT

V. Treatment

- ● Varicose veins can generally be treated on an outpatient basis.
- ● Self-care; patients should:
  - ○ Exercise
  - ○ Lose weight
  - ○ Avoid tight clothes
  - ○ Elevate legs
  - ○ Avoid long periods of standing or sitting
  - ○ Wear compression stockings all day; by squeezing the leg, these garments help the veins in the muscles move blood more efficiently.
- ● Varicose veins that develop during pregnancy will typically improve without medical treatment within 3 to 12 months following delivery.
- ● Additional options for severe cases not responding to self-care measures
  - ○ Sclerotherapy: small- and medium-sized varicose veins are injected with a solution (hypertonic saline or sodium tetradecyl sulfate) that scars and closes the veins

- ○ Catheter-assisted procedure for larger varicose veins: uses heat at the tip of a catheter as it is pulled out to collapse and seal a problem vein.

- ○ Removal of a long vein through a small incision

- ○ Removal of smaller varicose veins through a series of tiny skin punctures.

- ○ Possible complications of surgery: infection of incision made in groin crease, blood leaking and collecting outside of the blood vessels

- Refer the patient to a hospital for treatment if:

  - ○ Deep vein thrombosis (DVT) is diagnosed

  - ○ Uncontrolled bleeding occurs

  - ○ Infection requiring long-term therapy is found

  - ○ Surgical intervention is required (skin grafting)

  - ○ Therapy or testing cannot be accomplished in field

VI. Complications

- Hemorrhage within extremity
- New onset of dermatitis
- Blood clot (DVT)
- Bacterial skin infection
- Ulceration
- Worsening, chronic symptoms

References

Deep Vein Thrombosis. Wikipedia. en.wikipedia.org/wiki/Deep_vein_thrombosis

How to Prevent Varicose Veins. WikiHow. www.wikihow.com/Prevent-Varicose-Veins

Varicose Veins. eMedicineHealth.
   www.emedicinehealth.com/varicose_veins-health/article_em.htm

Varicose Veins. Mayo Clinic.
   www.mayoclinic.org/diseases-conditions/varicose-veins/basics/definition/con-20043474

Varicose Veins Exam. Clinical Exam. www.clinicalexam.com/pda/c_varicose_veins.htm

Figure 4.1 Normal and Varicose Veins. Source: National Heart, Lung, and Blood Institute; National Institutes of Health; U.S. Department of Health and Human Services / Public Domain, File:Varicose veins.jpg. Image at www.nhlbi.nih.gov/health/health-topics/topics/vv/causes.html

Figure 4.2 Skin Changes Commonly Seen in Varicose Veins. Source: Lakeland1999 / Wikimedia Commons / Public Domain. Image at commons.wikimedia.org/wiki/File:Leg_Before_1.jpg

Figure 4.3 Leg Ulcers. Source: Rfc1394 / Wikimedia Commons / Public Domain. Image at commons.wikimedia.org/wiki/File:Leg_ulcer.png

Figure 4.4 The Saphenofemoral Opening. Source: Henry Gray / Wikimedia Commons / Public Domain. Image at en.wikipedia.org/wiki/File:Great_saphenous_vein.png

Superficial Venous Thrombosis
By Andrea Wakim

Introduction

- Superficial veins lie relatively close to the surface of the body.
- Superficial venous thrombosis, also known as thrombophlebitis, is inflammation caused by a blood clot in a superficial vein in the upper or lower extremities.
- Risk factors include:
  - Family history
  - Damage to nearby veins
  - Varicose veins: enlarged, twisted, or inflamed veins that are sensitive to the touch
  - Hypercoagulable states: an abnormally increased tendency to form blood clots
  - Poor blood circulation

I. Basic Physiology

- A blood clot forms when platelets in the blood gather at a site of injury, form a plug, and release chemicals to begin forming the protein fibrin. Fibrin links with itself and forms the final mesh-like clot.
- The formation of blood clots (thrombosis) is often accompanied by phlebitis, or inflammation of the vein, hence the name thrombophlebitis.
- Superficial venous thrombosis occurs most frequently in the legs.

II. Clinical Signs and Symptoms

- Often occurs in varicose veins
- Red and inflamed cord under surface of skin
- Tenderness and pain in affected area
- Edema: swelling caused by fluid retention
- Pain is often more noticeable when standing or walking.
- Skin may turn a blue or purple color, often appearing in patches.
- Low-grade fever may develop.

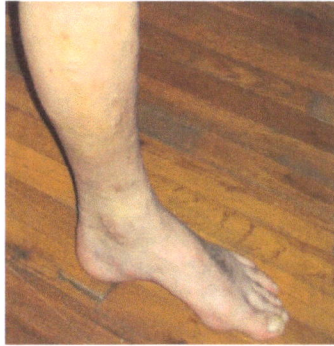

Figure 4.5 Varicose Veins in the Lower Leg.

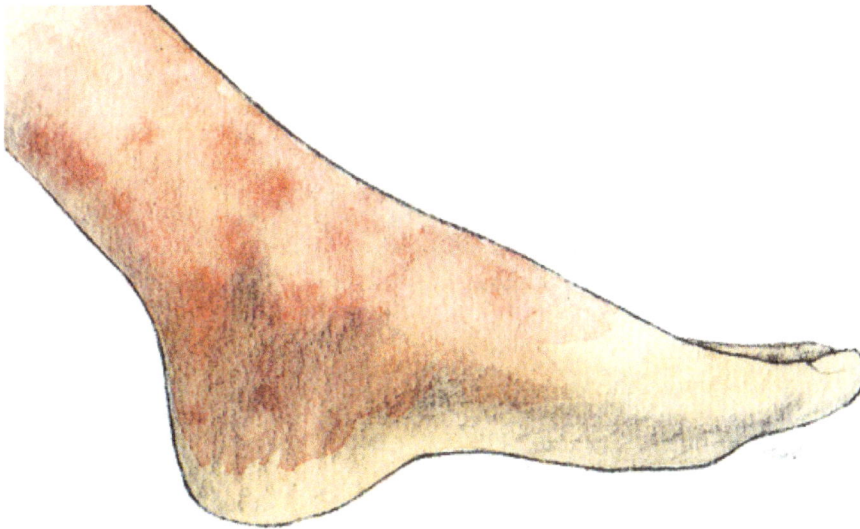

Figure 4.6 Blotchy and Inflamed Appearance of Superficial Venous Thrombosis.

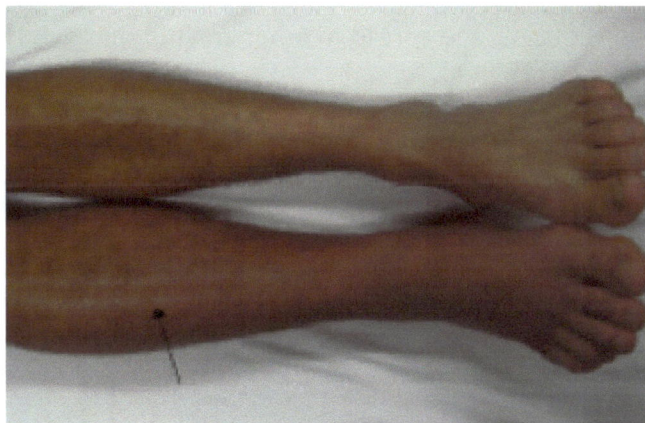

Figure 4.7 Swelling and Redness Characteristic of Venous Thrombosis.

III. Differential Diagnosis

- Can be confused with deep vein thrombosis (DVT), in which the clot forms in a deep vein as opposed to a superficial one.

  ○ Clots from DVT are more dangerous because they can travel to the lungs and block an artery, a painful and serious condition called a pulmonary embolism

  ○ The pain of superficial venous thrombosis should subside within about 2 weeks.

  ○ Symptoms of DVT are similar, but more severe, with longer lasting symptoms and pain.

  ○ Ultrasound of the affected area can be used to look for clots in deeper veins.

IV. Treatment

- Elevate affected leg (or area) regularly and apply heat.

- Encourage movement of area.

- Compression (tight) socks

- Anti-coagulants are typically not needed due to the benign nature of the condition, unless DVT is diagnosed.

- Creams and gels that are heparinoid-based, such as Hirudoid, may be used to improve circulation.

  ○ Gently apply 5–15 cm to the affected area up to 4 times a day.

  ○ Do not use the cream/gel on children under the age of 5, on broken, sensitive, or large areas of skin, or on any internal tissues.

V. Complications

- Complications can arise if the blood clot extends further up into the vein, joining a deep vein, resulting in DVT.

- Infection is rare but can occur and spread to other areas of the body. If so, antibiotics are needed.

- Superficial vein thrombosis can be recurrent and is occasionally a sign of a more severe condition, such as polyarteritis nodosa (uneven inflammation of artery walls) or cancer.

References

Definition of Hypercoagulable State. MedicineNet.com.
www.medterms.com/script/main/art.asp?articlekey=9240

Douketis, James D. Superficial Vein Thrombosis. Merck Manuals.
www.merckmanuals.com/professional/cardiovascular-disorders/peripheral-venous-disorders/superficial-venous-thrombosis

DVT and Thrombophlebitis. Mims.
www.mims.co.uk/deep-vein-thrombosis-dvt-thrombophlebitis/cardiovascular-system/article/882258

Hirudoid Cream/Gel. Net Doctor.
www.netdoctor.co.uk/skin-and-hair/medicines/hirudoid-cream.html

Moser, K.M., and Fedullo, P.F. Venous Thromboembolism: Three Simple Decisions. *Chest* 83, no. 117 (1983): 256.

Rosh, Adam J. Superficial Thrombophlebitis. Medscape.
emedicine.medscape.com/article/463256-overview#showall

Superficial Thrombophlebitis. Patient.co.uk. www.patient.co.uk/health/Phlebitis.htm

Thrombophlebitis. Mayo Clinic.
www.mayoclinic.com/health/thrombophlebitis/DS00223/DSECTION=symptoms

What Is Deep Vein Thrombosis. NIH: National Heart Lung and Blood Institute.
www.nhlbi.nih.gov/health/health-topics/topics/dvt/

What Is Edema? Medical News Today.
www.medicalnewstoday.com/articles/159111.php

Figure 4.5 Varicose Veins in the Lower Leg. Source: Lakeland1999 / Wikimedia Commons / Public Domain. Image at
upload.wikimedia.org/wikipedia/commons/0/01/Lower_leg_and_Foot_5_days_after.jpg

Figure 4.6 Blotchy and Inflamed Appearance of Superficial Venous Thrombosis. Source: Laura Gajewski, Medical illustrator.

Figure 4.7 Swelling and Redness Characteristic of Venous Thrombosis. Source: James Heilman, MD, File: Deep vein thrombosis of the right leg.jpg, CC-BY-SA-3.0/ GNU Free Documentation License. Image at
commons.wikimedia.org/wiki/Category:Deep_vein_thrombosis#mediaviewer/File:Deep_vein_thrombosis_of_the_right_leg.jpg

Chapter 5:

Other Cardiovascular Conditions

Lymphedema
By Evan Anderson

Introduction

- Lymphedema is swelling due to a blockage of the lymph vessels.
- Lymph vessels carry lymph fluid throughout the body.
- Lymph fluid collects bacteria, viruses, and waste products in order to rid them from the body.
- Common causes
  - Cancer
  - Infection
  - Scar tissue
  - Surgical removal of lymph nodes (often as part of mastectomy, removal of breast)
  - Inherited disorders

I. Clinical Signs and Symptoms

- Chronic swelling of one or more limbs
- Swelling may be partial, or may affect the entire limb
- Discomfort in the affected limb
- Recurring infections in the affected limb

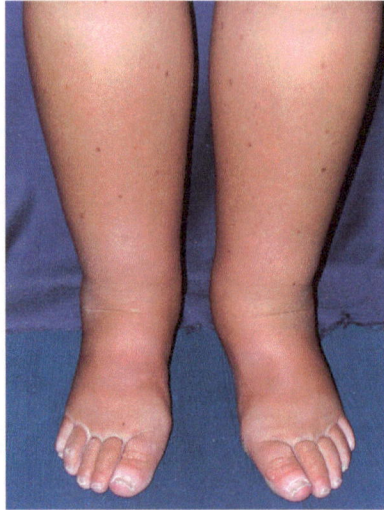

Figure 5.1 Bilateral Lymphedema in the Legs.

II. Treatment

- There is no cure for lymphedema; lifelong management is required.
- Therapy is targeted at increasing the flow of lymph in the affected limb. This includes:
  - ○ Any light exercise involving the affected limb.
  - ○ Compression of the affected limb; wrap tightly with a bandage, starting at the fingers or toes, and loosening the fit of the bandage as you move up the limb.
  - ○ Elevation of the affected limb
  - ○ Good skin care is vital to minimizing the naturally higher risk of infection seen in patients with lymphedema.

III. Complication

- Infection

References

Lymphedema. Mayo Clinic. www.mayoclinic.com/health/lymphedema/DS00609

McPhee, Stephen J., and Papadakis, Maxine A. (2008). *Current Medical Diagnosis and Treatment 2010* (49th ed.). New York: McGraw-Hill Medical.

Figure 5.1 Bilateral Lymphedema in the Legs. Source: Stephane Vignes, Jerome Bellanger / Wikimedia Commons / CC-BY-SA-2.0 / Public Domain. Image at commons.wikimedia.org/wiki/File:PIL.jpg

Hypertension
By Michael J. Cox

Introduction

- Hypertension is an all-encompassing term used to describe a sustained elevated blood pressure that puts a patient at risk for other health problems.

- Hypertension is the leading cause of stroke and is a major contributor to heart attack.

I. Pathophysiology

- Blood pressure (BP) is the force of blood pushing against arterial walls as the heart pumps it through the body.

- There is a variety of factors that can affect blood pressure; the most common are:

  ○ Water intake: reduced water intake can lead to dehydration. In response, the body begins using water from the bloodstream. Decreased water volume in circulation increases the viscosity (thickness) of blood and requires much more pressure to move it along.

  ○ Salt intake: too much dietary salt can exceed the kidneys' abilities, allowing salt to circulate in the bloodstream. Salt attracts more water into the bloodstream, thereby increasing blood volume and, consequently, blood pressure.

  ○ Hormone levels: various hormones can affect the constriction (closing/narrowing) or dilation (opening/widening) of blood vessels.

  ○ Smoking: can cause a narrowing of blood vessels, which increases vessel resistance

  ○ Obesity: the heart must pump harder to get more blood to the additional areas of body mass

  ○ Condition of kidneys, nervous system and blood vessels

- Risk of high blood pressure increases with the following:

  ○ Increasing age

  ○ African (black) heritage

  ○ High stress levels

  ○ Family history of hypertension and high blood pressure

  ○ Diabetes

II. Clinical Signs and Symptoms

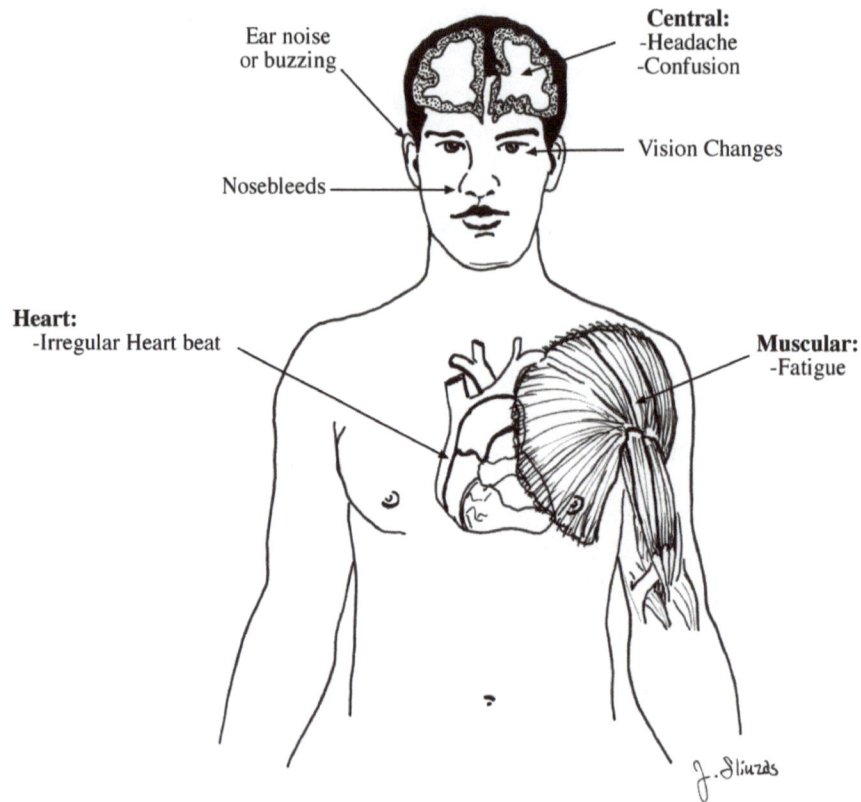

Figure 5.2 Possible Symptoms of Hypertension.

- Hypertension does not typically present with any signs or symptoms other than elevated blood pressure, which is why it is often considered a "silent" disease. However, some symptoms that may occur include:

  ○ Confusion

  ○ Fatigue

  ○ Headache

  ○ Irregular heartbeat

  ○ Nosebleeds

  ○ Vision changes

  ○ Ear noise or buzzing

- If symptoms are present, patients should receive immediate medical attention as the symptoms may be the signs of a complication of malignant hypertension, or dangerously high blood pressure.

III. Diagnostic Work-up

- Blood pressure is measured using a sphygmomanometer and is read in units of millimeters of mercury. The measurement consists of two numbers, written as a fraction.

  - For example: 120/80 mm Hg

  - The top number in the BP reading is your **systolic pressure**, the pressure on the arteries during a heartbeat. Normal systolic BP is below 120.

  - The bottom number in the BP reading is your **diastolic pressure**, the pressure on the arteries between beats, while the heart is relaxed. Normal diastolic BP is below 80.

- Hypertension can be categorized into different types:

  - **Primary hypertension**: called idiopathic (no known cause) or essential hypertension, affects 90–95% of hypertensive individuals, and is a combined systolic and diastolic hypertension. This type of hypertension typically results from a combination of genetic and environmental factors.

  - **Secondary hypertension**: caused by altered blood flow, secondary to another primary disease—typically other kidney or endocrine disorders

  - **Isolated systolic hypertension**: characterized by elevated systolic blood pressure and normal diastolic blood pressure. Isolated systolic hypertension is an expression of increased cardiac output, increased arterial resistance, or a combination of the two.

  - **Malignant hypertension**: a rapid and sudden development of extremely high blood pressure with diastolic readings often exceeding 140 mm Hg. Individuals who have had kidney failure or renal hypertension are at the highest risk for developing malignant hypertension.

  - **Note**: a single, elevated BP reading does not mean a person has hypertension. Diagnosis requires a documented increased BP over two or more different occasions.

Table 5.1 Classification of Blood Pressure in Adults

Category	Systolic (mm Hg)	Diastolic (mm Hg)
Normal	<120	<80
Prehypertension	120–139	80–89
Stage 1 hypertension	140–159	90–99
Stage 2 hypertension	≥160	≥100

IV. Treatment

- The primary goal of treatment is to reduce blood pressure to avoid any related complications. Medications include the following:

  o Alpha blockers: relax muscles and help smaller blood vessels remain open by preventing the hormone norepinephrine from constricting the walls of arteries and veins.

  o Angiotensin-converting enzyme (ACE) inhibitors: prevent enzymes from producing angiotensin II, which normally triggers the cardiovascular system to narrow blood vessels and release hormones that raise blood pressure.

  o Angiotensin receptor blockers (ARBs): block angiotensin II receptors, which helps relax blood vessels and makes it easier for the heart to pump blood.

  o Beta blockers: block the effects of the hormone epinephrine, which normally increases heart rate and constricts blood vessels.

  o Calcium channel blockers: prevent calcium from entering muscle cells in the heart and blood vessels; relax and widen blood vessels.

  o Central alpha agonists: prevent the brain from signaling the nervous system to increase heart rate and constrict blood vessels.

  o Diuretics: force the kidneys to excrete more sodium into the urine, which draws water from the blood with it. This decreases fluid in the vessels, reducing pressure on arterial walls.

  o Renin inhibitors: prevent kidneys from secreting renin, an enzyme that eventually leads to the production of angiotensin II.

  o Vasodilators: work directly on muscles in the walls of arteries to prevent constriction so that blood can flow more easily through them.

- In addition to prescribed medication, patients are encouraged to make lifestyle changes to help prevent progression of the disease. Recommendations include:
  - Eating a "heart-healthy" diet with lots of water and dietary fiber.
  - Regular daily exercise
  - Quit smoking.
  - Limit alcohol consumption.
  - Limit sodium consumption (less than 1,500 mg daily).
  - Reduce stress.
  - Maintain a healthy body weight—dieting if necessary.
- **Compelling indications**
  - Describes high-risk hypertension, as in patients with diabetes mellitus or kidney disease
  - After an initial medication is selected, the patient should be informed of side effects and the need for compliance.
  - Treatment should start at a low dose unless patient has stage 2 hypertension (≥160 mm Hg systolic BP or ≥100 mm Hg diastolic BP).
  - Follow-up visits should be scheduled at 4–6 week intervals. If an apparent but incomplete response is demonstrated, a second agent should be added.
  - Combinations of ACE Inhibitors, ARBs, or beta blockers with a calcium channel blocker or diuretic have demonstrated the greatest efficacy.

Table 5.2 Typical Initial Prescription for Hypertensive Patients

BP Class	Systolic BP (mm Hg)	Diastolic BP (mm Hg)	Initial Drug Therapy (without compelling indications)	Initial Drug Therapy (with compelling indications)
Pre-hypertension	120–139	80–89	Lifestyle modification only	Drugs for compelling indication
Stage 1 hypertension	140–159	90–99	Thiazide-type diuretics	Drugs for compelling indication + diuretic, ACE inhibitor, ARB, beta blocker or calcium channel blocker as needed
Stage 2 Hypertension	≥160	≥100	Two-drug combination (Thiazide-type diuretic + ACE Inhibitor)	Drugs for compelling indication + diuretic, ACE inhibitor, ARB, beta blocker or calcium channel blocker as needed

###

Table 5.3 Recommended Medication for Adults (Age ≥18) without Compelling Indications

Patient Characteristic	Step 1	Step 2	Step 3	Step 4: Resistant Hypertension
<55 years old and non-black	ACE Inhibitor, ARB, or beta blocker	ACE Inhibitor, ARB or beta blocker + calcium channel blocker or diuretic	ACE Inhibitor, ARB or beta blocker + calcium blocker + diuretic	Step 3 + alpha blocker or diuretic
≥55 years old or black (any age)	Calcium channel blocker or diuretic	Calcium channel blocker or diuretic + ACE Inhibitor, ARB or beta blocker	ACE Inhibitor, ARB or beta blocker + calcium channel blocker + diuretic	Step 3 + alpha blocker or diuretic

###

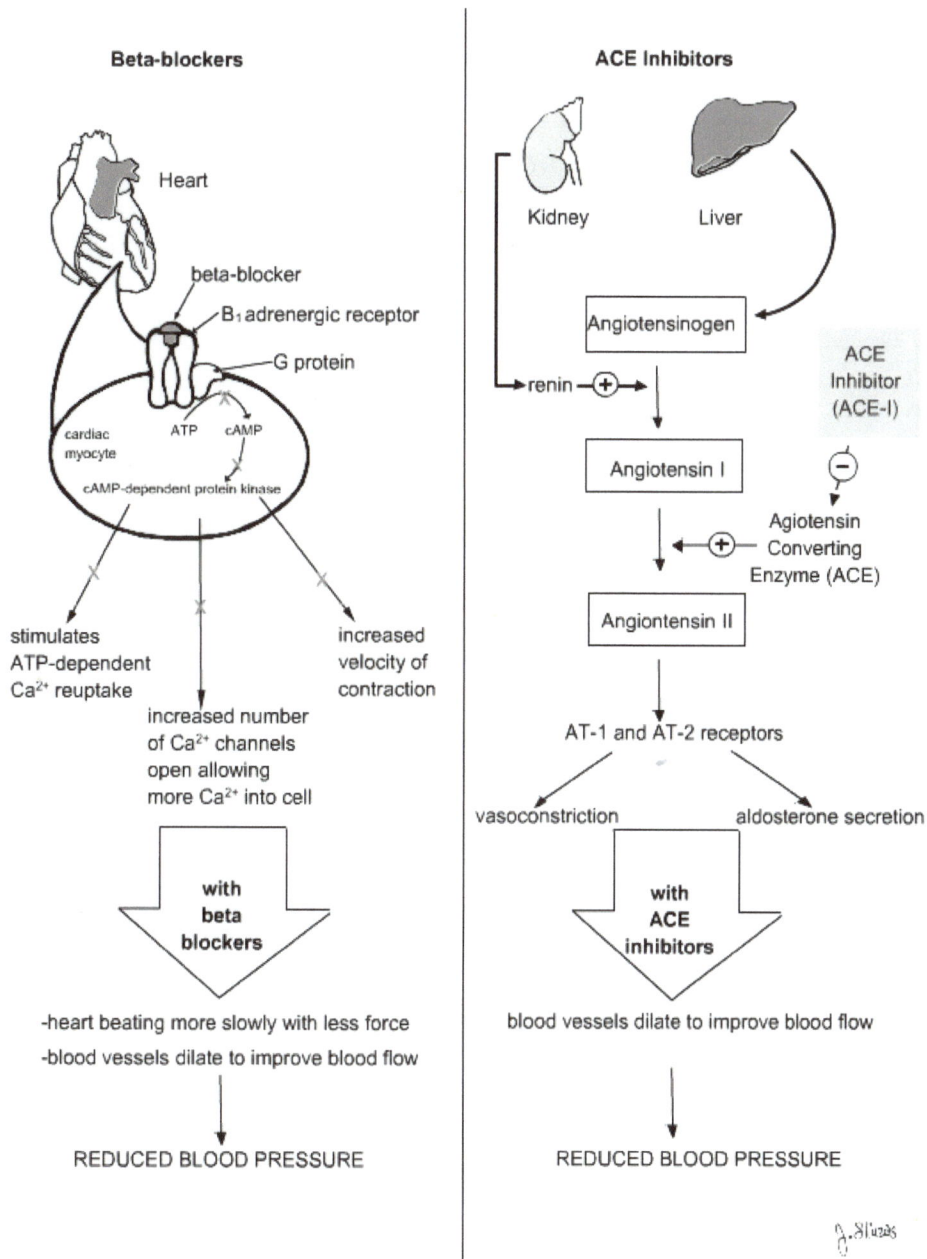

Figure 5.3 Actions of Beta-blockers and ACE Inhibitors.

Table 5.4 Antihypertensive Agents and Adverse Effects

Drug Type	Drug Name	Adverse Effects
Alpha blockers	Prazosin, Terazosin, Doxazosin	Syncope (fainting) with first dose Postural hypotension Dizziness Palpitations Headache Weakness Drowsiness Sexual dysfunction Anticholinergic effects (e.g., constipation, dry mouth, blurred vision, decreased urination) Urinary incontinence Note: first-dose effects may be less with doxazosin
ACE inhibitors	Benazepril, Captopril, Enalapril, Fosinopril, Lisinopril, Moexipril, Perindopril, Quinapril, Ramipril, Trandolapril	Cough Hypotension Dizziness Kidney dysfunction High potassium levels Swelling of deep layers of the skin Taste alteration Rash (more frequent with captopril) Rarely, protein in urine Blood dyscrasia (blood disease) *Do not use in pregnant patients.*

Drug Type	Drug Name	Adverse Effects
ARBs	Candesartan cilexitil*, Eprosartan*, Irbesartan*, Losartan*, Olmesartan*, Telmisartan*, Valsartan*	High potassium levels Metabolic acidosis Gynecomastia (swelling of the breast tissue in males)
Beta blockers	Acebutolol, Atenolol, Betaxolol, Bisoprolol*, Carvedilol, Labetalol, Metoprolol, Nadolol, Penbutolol, Pindolol, Propranolol, Timolol	Bronchospasm Fatigue Sleep disturbance and nightmares Bradycardia and atrioventricular block Worsening of congestive heart failure Cold extremities Gastrointestinal disturbances Erectile dysfunction Decreased HDL cholesterol Rare blood dyscrasias
Calcium channel blockers	Diltiazem, Verapamil, Amlodipine, Felodipine, Isradipine, Nicardipine, Nifedipine, Nisoldipine	Edema Headache Bradycardia Gastrointestinal disturbances Dizziness AV block Congestive heart failure Urinary frequency

Drug Type	Drug Name	Adverse Effects
Central alpha agonists	Clonidine, Guanabenz, Guanfacine, Methyldopa	Sedation Dry mouth Sexual dysfunction Headache Bradyarrhythmias Side effects may be less with Guanfacine. Contact dermatitis may develop with clonidine patch. Methyldopa also causes hepatitis, hemolytic anemia, fever
Diuretics (thiazide type)	Hydrochlorothiazide, Chlorthalidone, Metolazone, Indapamide	Decreased potassium, magnesium, and sodium Increased calcium, uric acid, glucose, LDL cholesterol and triglycerides Rash Erectile dysfunction
Loop diuretics	Furosemide, Ethacrynic acid, Bumetanide, Torsemide	Same as for thiazides, but with a higher risk of excessive urination and electrolyte imbalances. Increases calcium excretion
Renin inhibitors	Aliskiren*	Swelling of deep layers of skin Hypotension High potassium levels

Drug Type	Drug Name	Adverse Effects
Direct vasodilators	Hydralazine, Minoxidil	Gastrointestinal disturbances
		Tachycardia
		Headache
		Nasal congestion
		Rash
		Lupus erythematosus-like syndrome (causing lupus-like symptoms, e.g., joint pain, muscle pain, fever, etc.)
		Tachycardia
		Fluid retention
		Headache
		Excessive hairiness
		Pericardial effusion (abnormal build-up of excess fluid between the pericardium and heart)
		Thrombocytopenia (low blood platelet count)
May be combined with hydrochlorothiazide (HCTZ)		

V. Complications

- Progression of hypertension can lead to a number of other disease processes, including:
  - Heart attack or stroke
  - Aneurysm (a bulge or "ballooning" in the wall of an artery)
  - Heart failure
  - Weakened and narrowed renal blood vessels
  - Thickened, narrowed or torn blood vessels in the eyes
  - Vision loss
  - Peripheral artery disease

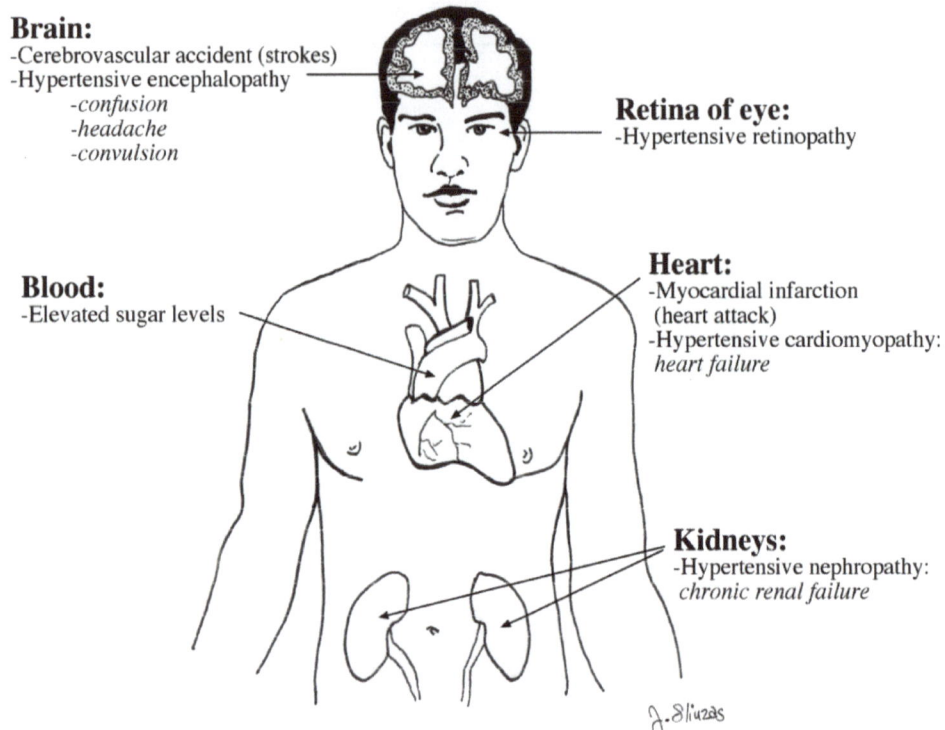

Brain:
-Cerebrovascular accident (strokes)
-Hypertensive encephalopathy
     -confusion
     -headache
     -convulsion

Retina of eye:
-Hypertensive retinopathy

Blood:
-Elevated sugar levels

Heart:
-Myocardial infarction
 (heart attack)
-Hypertensive cardiomyopathy:
 heart failure

Kidneys:
-Hypertensive nephropathy:
 chronic renal failure

Figure 5.4 Main Complications of Persistent High Blood Pressure.

VI. Prevention

- Since hypertension is commonly a result of environmental factors, there are many things even a genetically predisposed individual can do to help reduce risk, including:

   ○ Maintaining a healthy weight

   ○ Engaging in regular exercise

   ○ Limiting salt intake

   ○ Limiting alcohol consumption

   ○ Reducing stress

- Certain dietary components may also play a role in prevention. Diets rich in the following dietary supplements have shown benefits:

   ○ Potassium

   ○ Calcium

   ○ Magnesium

   ○ Fish oil (omega-3 fatty acids)

   ○ Garlic

References

Aronow, Wilbert S. Treatment of Hypertension in Older Adults. *Geriatrics and Aging* 11, no. 8 (2008): 457–463.

Chobanian, A.V., Bakris, G.L., Black, H.R., et al., for the Joint National Committee on Prevention, Detection, Evaluation, and Treatment of High Blood Pressure. National Heart, Lung, and Blood Institute. Seventh report of the Joint National Committee on Prevention, Detection, Evaluation, and Treatment of High Blood Pressure. *Hypertension* 42 (2003): 1206–1252.

Häggström, Mikael. Main Complications of Persistent High Blood Pressure. Wikimedia Commons. commons.wikimedia.org/wiki/File:Main_complications_of_persistent_high_blood_pressure.svg

High Blood Pressure (Hypertension). Mayo Clinic. www.mayoclinic.com/health/high-blood-pressure/DS00100

High Blood Pressure Treatments: Lifestyle Changes and Medications. WebMD. www.webmd.com/hypertension-high-blood-pressure/guide/hypertension-treatment-overview

Hypertension. PubMed Health. www.ncbi.nlm.nih.gov/pubmedhealth/PMH0001502/

McCance, Kathryn L., and Huether, Sue E. (2006). *Pathophysiology: The Biologic Basis for Disease in Adults and Children*. St. Louis, MO: Elsevier Mosby.

McPhee, Stephen J., and Papadakis, Maxine A. (2008). *Current Medical Diagnosis and Treatment 2010* (49th ed.). New York: McGraw-Hill Medical.

Figures 5.2–5.4 Source: Jana Sliuzas, Medical illustrator.

Infective Endocarditis

By Evan Anderson

Introduction

- Endocarditis is an inflammation of the endocardium.
- The endocardium is the layer of tissue that forms the innermost lining of the chambers and valves of the heart.
- There are two types of infective endocarditis:
  - Infections caused by bacteria
  - More rarely, fungal infections
- Uncommon in individuals without preexisting heart problems
- Risk factors:
  - Artificial heart valves
  - Damaged heart valves
  - Congenital heart disease
  - History of rheumatic heart disease
  - Preexisting organic heart lesion
  - Intravenous drug abuse

I. Clinical Signs and Symptoms

- Positive blood cultures for bacteria in the bloodstream
- Positive echocardiogram findings
  - Distinct, abnormal outgrowths
  - Myocardial abscesses
  - Problems with prosthetic (artificial) valve
  - New or changing abnormal heart sounds
- Fever: virtually all patients with endocarditis have fever to some extent
- Vascular problems
  - Stroke, or other blood flow disruptions in the body

○ Aneurysm (a bulge or "ballooning" in the wall of an artery)

○ Death of lung tissue due to lack of blood supply

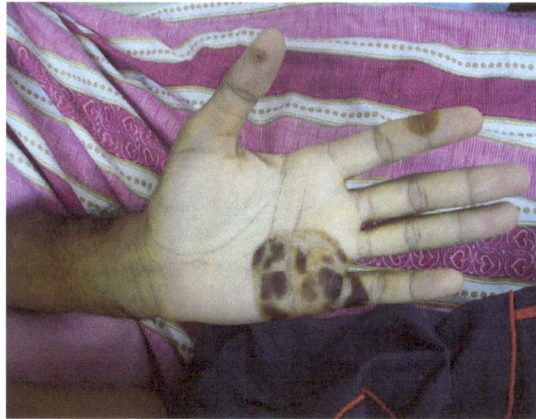

Figure 5.5 Osler's Nodes in Patient Diagnosed with Bacterial Endocarditis.

● Immunologic findings

    ○ Osler's nodes: painful, red, raised lesions located on hands or feet (Figure 5.5)

    ○ Roth spots: retinal hemorrhages with a white center (Figure 5.6)

    ○ Blood in urine

    ○ Diarrhea

    ○ Fatigue

    ○ Cough

    ○ Shortness of breath

    ○ Tenderness of the spleen

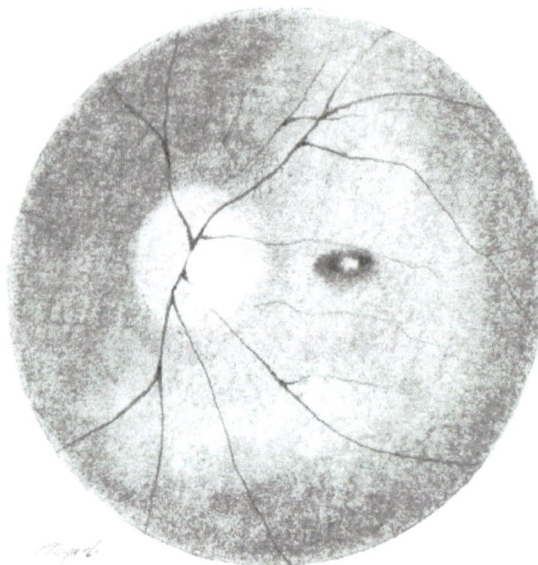

Figure 5.6 Roth Spot on the Retina.

II. Treatment

- **While waiting for culture results:**
  - If the patient appears to be seriously ill, start vancomycin after obtaining the blood for cultures.
  - Then switch to the appropriate drug after the results come back.
  - Most cases of infective endocarditis are due to *Staphylococcus* and will respond to vancomycin.
- Once culture results are obtained, alter drug therapy based on infective organism.

Table 5.5 Dosing Guidelines for Vancomycin in Infective Endocarditis with Unconfirmed Pathogen

Drug Name	Dosage
Vancomycin	1 g IV every 12 hours

Table 5.6 Treatment for Infectious Endocarditis Caused by Streptococci

Drug Name	Dosage
Penicillin G	2–3 million units IV every 4 hours for 4 weeks
	OR
Ceftriaxone	2 g IV or IM once daily for 4 weeks
	OR
Vancomycin	15 mg/kg IV every 12 hours for 4 weeks
Note: If streptococci are relatively resistant to penicillin, penicillin G may be supplemented with gentamicin, 1 mg/kg IV every 8 hours	

Table 5.7 Treatment for Infectious Endocarditis Caused by Enterococci

Drug Name	Dosage
Penicillin G	3–4 million units IV every 4 hours for 4–6 weeks
	PLUS
Gentamicin	1 mg/kg IV every 8 hours for 4–6 weeks

Table 5.8 Treatment for Infectious Endocarditis Caused by Staphylococci

Drug Name	Dosage
Nafcillin	1.5–2 g IV every 4 hours for 6 weeks
	OR
Oxacillin	1.5–2 g IV every 4 hours for 6 weeks
	OR

Drug Name	Dosage
Cefazolin	2 g IV every 8 hours
	OR
Vancomycin	15 mg/kg IV every 12 hours

Table 5.9 Treatment for Infectious Endocarditis Caused by HACEK* Organisms

Drug Name	Dosage
Ceftriaxone	2 g IV every 24 hours for 4 weeks
* Gram-negative bacteria including *Haemophilus* species, *Actinobacillus*, *Cardiobacterium*, *Eikenella* and *Kingella* species	

- **Aftercare**
  - If condition is clearly resolving, gradually decrease antibiotic dosage.
  - Antibiotics will likely need to be continued for at least 6 weeks.
  - Once condition has resolved, do not decrease past the minimum dosage for a full week to prevent antibiotic resistance.
  - If condition is not improving, obtain another blood culture.
  - The patient may need surgery if infection is causing strokes, heart failure develops due to a damaged valve, there is severe organ damage, or persistent infections occur.
  - Causes of persistent fever include:
    - Abscess in the muscle tissue of the heart, or secondary abscess
    - Multiple infections
    - A blockage of a blood vessel
    - Drug reactions

III. Complications

- Stroke

- Organ damage due to blood clot

- Heart failure

- Arrhythmia

- Abscess

References

Endocarditis. Mayo Clinic.
www.mayoclinic.org/diseases-conditions/endocarditis/basics/definition/con-20022403

Endocarditis. PubMed Health. www.ncbi.nlm.nih.gov/pubmedhealth/PMH0001701/

McPhee, Stephen J., and Papadakis, Maxine A. (2008). *Current Medical Diagnosis and Treatment 2010* (49th ed.). New York: McGraw-Hill Medical.

White-centred Retinal Haemorrhages. NIH: National Center for Biotechnology Information.
www.ncbi.nlm.nih.gov/pmc/articles/PMC2361020/

Figure 5.5 Osler's Nodes in Patient Diagnosed with Bacterial Endocarditis. Source: Roberto J. Galindo / Wikimedia Commons / CC-BY-SA-3.0 / GNU Free Documentation License. Image at
commons.wikimedia.org/wiki/File:Osler_Nodules_Hand.jpg

Figure 5.6 Roth Spot on the Retina. Source: Laura Gajewski, Medical illustrator.

Abdominal Aortic Aneurysms and Acute Aortic Dissections

By Evan Anderson

Introduction

- An abdominal aortic aneurysm (AAA) is a condition in which the abdominal aorta becomes abnormally large (Figure 5.7.)

- The abdominal aorta is the main artery that supplies blood to the abdomen, pelvis, and legs.

- Abdominal aortic aneurysms vary only by their size and location.

- The larger the aneurysm, the greater the risk of rupture.

- AAAs are most likely to occur in males over the age of 65.

- An acute aortic dissection (AAD) is different from AAA.

- AAD is a tear through a layer of the aortic vessel that creates a false channel (Figure 5.8).

- AAD can occur in the ascending aorta and affect the great vessels.

  - This can also lead to cardiac tamponade (pressure on the heart from fluid build-up in the pericardial space).

- AAD most often occurs in the descending aorta.

  - The false channel can extend to the iliac arteries and beyond.

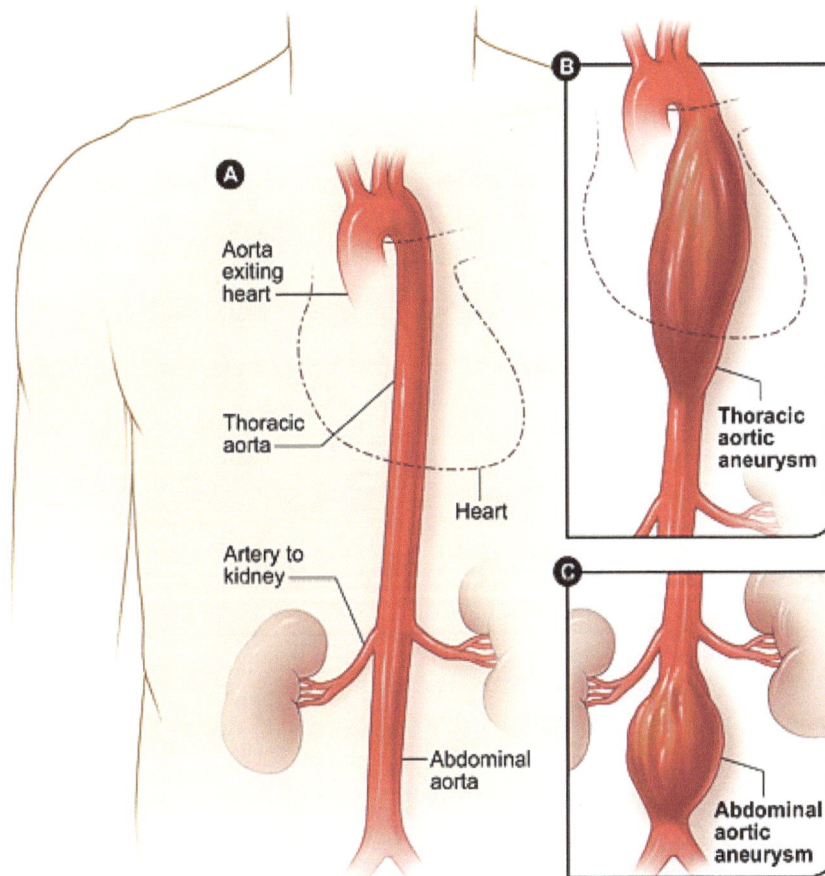

Figure 5.7 Aortic Aneurysm. (A) Normal aorta image. (B) Thoracic aortic aneurysm (less common than abdominal aneurysm). (C) Abdominal aortic aneurysm, below the arteries that supply blood to the kidneys.

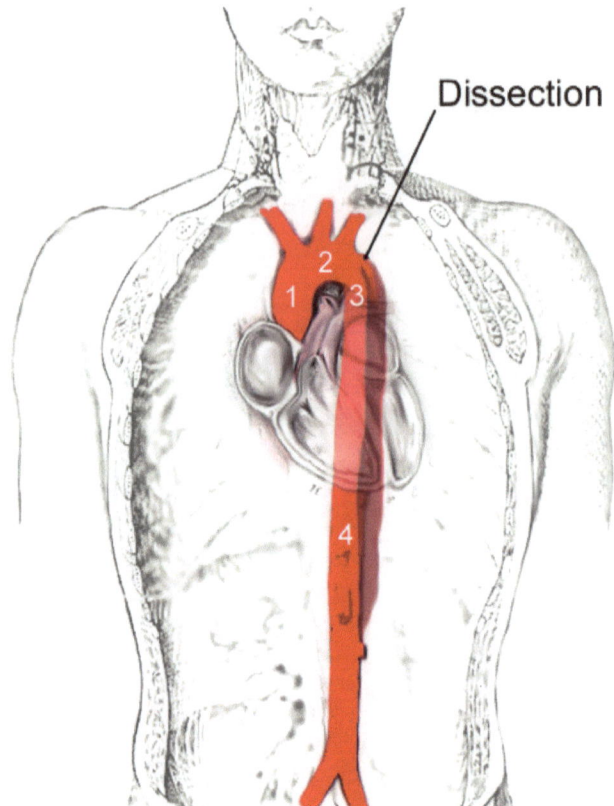

Figure 5.8 Acute Aortic Dissection. Note the dissection originated between markers 2 and 3 and the channel has extended beyond marker 4.

I. Basic Physiology

- In a healthy heart, the wall of the aorta is elastic, adjusting to blood flow. If the wall is damaged or weakened, it may begin to bulge outward, tear, or dissect.

- Risk factors:
  - Family history
  - Aging
  - Smoking
  - High blood pressure
  - Atherosclerosis (hardening of the arteries)
  - Infection in the aorta

II. Clinical Signs and Symptoms

- **AAA**: pulsating feeling near navel (note: this can be a normal finding in thin individuals)

- Many abdominal aneurysms do not cause any symptoms.
- **AAD:** sudden onset of chest pain with tearing or ripping quality extending to the mid-back
- Hypertension
  - Blood pressure may be 20 mm Hg different between arms; compare radial pulses.
  - Use higher blood pressure to guide medication therapy.
- Mid-abdominal pain
- Lower back pain
- Numbness or pain to lower extremities
- Monitor for abrupt onset of sharp, tearing pain, which may indicate rupture of aneurysm.
  - Patient may subsequently display signs of hypovolemic shock (condition in which the heart is unable to pump enough blood to the body due to severe blood and fluid loss).
  - Vital signs may remain normal if the rupture is a slow leak.

III. Diagnostic Work-up

- If AAA or AAD are suspected, an X-ray or ultrasound can be used to confirm diagnosis.
  - May show widened mediastinum
- CT scan is commonly used to diagnose AAD in stable patients.
- An ultrasound can be an effective method to measure the size of an AAA.
- Dilation of the artery is typically defined as a 50% increase over normal diameter (about 3 cm).

IV. Differential Diagnoses

- Appendicitis
- Cholelithiasis (gallstones)
- Diverticular disease
- Gastritis and peptic ulcer disease
- Large bowel obstruction
- Myocardial infarction
- Myocarditis
- Pancreatitis
- Small bowel obstruction
- Urinary tract infection (in women)

V. Treatment

- Can be managed medically or with surgery, depending on parameters including size and potential for rupture.

- Initial management includes pain control and decreasing heart rate (HR) and blood pressure (BP) to prevent extension of AAA or AAD.

  ○ Target BP and HR vary by surgeon or physician preference.

  ○ A reasonable HR target is 60–80 beats/minute.

  ○ A reasonable systolic blood pressure (SBP) target is about 120 mm Hg.

- Beta-blockers have been shown to decrease expansion rate of small aneurysms.

- Choose an agent to lower heart rate (60–80/minute) and lower SBP to near 120 mm Hg

  ○ Beta-blockers

    ▶ Esmolol (Brevibloc)

      ▷ Bolus 1 mg/kg IVP over 30 seconds, then

      ▷ 0.15–0.3 mg/kg/minute IV infusion, titrate as needed to target BP (about 120 mm Hg)

    ▶ Labetolol (Trandate)

      ▷ 20 mg IV over 2 minutes initially, then 40–80 mg IV every 10 minutes; do not exceed 300 mg.

  ○ Vasodilator may also be used (does not affect HR)

    ▶ Nitroprusside (Nitropress, Nipride) guidelines and considerations:

      ▷ Initiate at 0.3 mcg/kg/minute and titrate by 0.5 mcg/kg/minute increments.

      ▷ Usual range is 3–4 mcg/kg/minute.

      ▷ Do not exceed 10 mcg/kg/minute.

      ▷ Monitor BP every 5 minutes (preferred) or with arterial line.

      ▷ Patient BP may respond abruptly to unpredictable threshold dose.

      ▷ Protect medication from light.

- Large (>5–6 cm), rapidly growing, or leaking aneurysms require surgical intervention, as do aortic dissections.

  ○ Aorta may be repaired surgically by a thoracic surgeon in an open procedure or stented via an endovascular approach.

  ○ A dissection involving the pericardium and great vessels may require multiple surgeons, including:

    ▶ Thoracic surgeon

> ▶ Cardiac surgeon
- Aftercare
  - ○ Follow-up checks with ultrasound or radiographs are recommended every 3 months during the first year following diagnosis, and every 6 months thereafter.
  - ○ Control hypertension and other risk factors

VI. Complications

- Blood clots
- Stroke
- Heart attack
- Kidney failure
- Aortic rupture
- Hypovolemic shock
- Exsanguination (extreme hemorrhage)

References

Abdominal Aortic Aneurysm. Mayo Clinic. www.mayoclinic.com/health/abdominal-aortic-aneurysm/ds01194

Aortic Dissection. Medscape. emedicine.medscape.com/article/2062452-overview

McPhee, Stephen J., and Papadakis, Maxine A. (2008). *Current Medical Diagnosis and Treatment 2010* (49th ed.). New York: McGraw-Hill Medical.

Rahimi, Saum A. Abdominal Aortic Aneurysm. Medscape. emedicine.medscape.com/article/1979501-overview

Figure 5.7 Aortic Aneurysm. Source: National Institutes of Health / Wikimedia Commons / Public Domain. Image at commons.wikimedia.org/wiki/File:Aortic_aneurysm.jpg

Figure 5.8 Acute Aortic Dissection. Source: Fvasconcellos; JHeuser / Wikimedia Commons / CC-BY-SA-3.0 / GNU Free Documentation License. Image at commons.wikimedia.org/wiki/File:AoDissekt_scheme_StanfordB_en.png

Peripheral Artery Disease

By Marian M. Houtman

Introduction

- Peripheral artery disease (PAD) is a common circulatory problem in which narrowed arteries reduce blood flow to the extremities (arms and legs).

- Also called peripheral vascular disease (PVD)

- Blood flow is not enough to keep up with the body's demand.

- Decreased blood flow causes leg pain when walking; this is called "intermittent claudication."

- PAD also is a sign of widespread fatty deposits (plaque) in the arteries (a condition called atherosclerosis, or "hardening of the arteries"), which leads to decreased blood supply to the brain and heart.

- Less commonly, PAD can be caused by trauma, inflammation, or radiation.

- Risk factors

  - Smoking

  - Diabetes

  - Obesity (body mass index >30)

  - High blood pressure (≥140/90 mm Hg)

  - High cholesterol (240 milligrams per deciliter or 6.2 millimoles per liter)

  - Increasing age (≥50 years)

  - Family history of PAD

  - High levels of homocysteine, a normal amino acid found in the body that helps build and maintain tissue, but at a high level, increases risk of PAD.

  - People who smoke and have diabetes are at the highest risk for PAD due to reduced blood flow.

I. Clinical Signs and Symptoms

- Mild or no symptoms

- Mild to severely debilitating cramping in the hip, thigh, and/or calf following activity or walking

- Temperature change (cool to the touch) in affected leg

- Sores that do not heal on affected leg, foot, or toes
- Affected extremity has change in color
- Loss of hair, slow growth of nails
- Shiny skin
- Weakened or no pulse
- Erectile dysfunction in men
- As disease progresses, sleep disturbance related to pain that is only relieved by getting up and moving legs

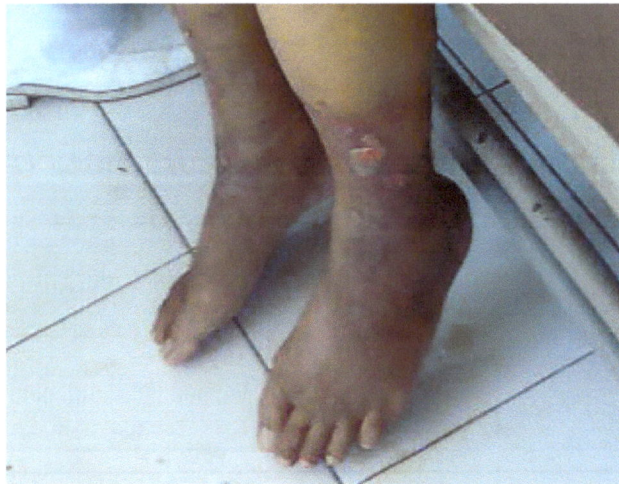

Figure 5.9 Sores, Skin Color Changes, and Hair Loss on the Legs Caused by PAD.

II. Diagnostic Work-up

- Weak or absent pulses
- Bruits: whooshing sound heard with stethoscope when listening over arteries
- Non-healing wound(s) on extremities
- Decreased blood pressure in affected extremity
- Shiny skin, lack of hair
- Lab tests: cholesterol level
- Ankle brachial pressure index (ABPI)
  - ○ Have the patient exercise (walk, treadmill).
  - ○ Take blood pressure on ankle and arm.
  - ○ Use blood pressure cuff and ultrasound (Doppler) and compare results.

○ The greater the blood pressure difference, the more severe the disease.

○ In a normal patient, the pressure at the ankle is slightly higher than at the elbow.

○ The ankle brachial pressure index is the ratio of the highest ankle to brachial artery pressure; an ABPI of greater than 0.9 is considered normal.

○ Greater than 1.3 is considered abnormal and suggests hardening of the arteries.

● If no other conditions are affecting the arteries of the legs, the ABPI ratios can be used to identify the nature and severity of PAD, and the best management of various types of leg ulcers. See Table 5.10.

○ Doppler-ultrasound can help determine areas of decreased blood flow.

○ If possible to refer patient to appropriate facility, angiography: dye is injected for doctor to view blood flow in the arteries with use of imaging magnetic resonance angiography (MRA) or computerized tomography angiography (CTA)

Table 5.10 Interpretation of Ankle Brachial Pressure Index (ABPI)

ABPI Value	Interpretation	Action	Nature of Ulcers, if Present
>1.2	Abnormal: vessel hardening from PAD	Refer routinely	Venous ulcer: full compression bandaging
1.0–1.2	Normal range	None	
0.9–1.0	Acceptable		
0.8–0.9	Some arterial disease	Manage risk factors	
0.5–0.8	Moderate arterial disease	Routine specialist referral	Mixed ulcers: use reduced compression bandaging
<0.5	Severe arterial disease	Urgent specialist referral	Arterial ulcers: no compression bandaging used

III. Treatment

● Goals are to manage symptoms and reduce the progression of disease. Quitting tobacco, eating healthily, and exercising can successfully treat PAD.

- Cholesterol-lowering drugs: "statins" (examples: Lipitor, Lescol, Mevacor, Prevachol, Crestor, Zocor, Livalo)

- Blood pressure-reducing medications (e.g., acebutolol, atenolol, betaxolol, bisoprolol, carteolol)

- Blood sugar control medications (e.g., acarbose, chlorpropamide, glimepiride, insulin, metformin)

- Medications to reduce potential for blood clotting

- Symptom relief medication

- Lifestyle changes

  - Quit smoking

  - Low salt, low fat diet

  - Exercise daily

  - Avoid cold medications

  - Schedule routine foot check

- Angioplasty surgery (femoral bypass graft)

Table 5.11 Pharmaceutical Treatment Options for PAD

Drug Classification	Drug Name	Dose (Adult)	Frequency	Comments
Hemorrheologic agent (xanthine)	**Pentoxifylline** (Trental)	400 mg	3 times daily	Action of drug not understood, but believed to improve blood flow by decreasing thickness of blood cells.
Antiplatelet	**Cilostazol** (Pletal)	100 mg	Twice a day, 30 minutes before a meal or 2 hours following breakfast and dinner	Prevents platelets from clumping together. Expands the blood vessels. Do not use if patient has congestive heart failure
Nonsteroidal anti-inflammatory	**Aspirin**	325–500 mg	Every 3 hours	Antiplatelet agents prevent clots from forming.
Antiplatelet	**Ticlopidine**	250 mg	Twice a day	Antiplatelet agents prevent clots from forming.

Drug Classification	Drug Name	Dose (Adult)	Frequency	Comments
Antiplatelet	**Clopidogrel**	75 mg	Daily with or without food	Antiplatelet agents prevent clots from forming.
Anticoagulant	**Heparin**	Dose adjusted for each patient on basis of laboratory test.		
Anticoagulant	**Warfarin** (Coumadin)	5–10 mg/day	For 4–5 days then lab test	Dose determined by international normalized ratio or prothrombin time
Anticoagulant	**Enoxaparin** (Lovenox)	1 mg/kg subcutaneously (SC) every 12 hours or 1.5 mg/kg SC once a day	Every 12 hours	For DVT or pulmonary embolism for outpatients
Thrombolytics				Powerful drugs injected into blocked artery under angiographic guidance in a hospital setting

###

IV. Complications

- Critical limb ischemia (CLI): blood flow to extremity is severely decreased, leading to open sores, infection, gangrene (dying tissue) and possible amputation
- Stroke or heart attack if major arteries to the brain or heart are impacted by plaque in vessels

References

Ankle brachial pressure index. Wikipedia. en.wikipedia.org/wiki/Ankle_brachial_pressure_index

Peripheral Artery Disease (PAD).
   Mayo Clinic. www.mayoclinic.com/health/peripheral-arterial disease/DS00537

Statins. MedicineNet. www.medicinenet.com/statins/article.htm

Figure 5.9 Sores, Skin Color Changes, and Hair Loss on the Legs Caused by PAD. Wikimedia Commons.
   Source: Wfnicdao / Wikimedia Commons / Public Domain. Image at
   en.wikipedia.org/wiki/File:Pvd002.jpg

Raynaud's Phenomenon
By Evan Anderson

Introduction

- Raynaud's phenomenon is a condition that causes lack of blood flow to the extremities.
- Two types
  - **Raynaud's disease (primary)**: mild, intermittent attacks of Raynaud's symptoms with an unknown cause. Symptoms typically appear equally on both sides of hands or feet.
  - **Raynaud's phenomenon (secondary)**: intermittent attacks of Raynaud's symptoms secondary to an underlying condition. Symptoms may be most noticeable in one hand or even one or two fingers.
- May affect fingers, toes, ears, or nose
- Risk factors
  - Aging
  - Smoking
  - More common in females and individuals living in colder climates

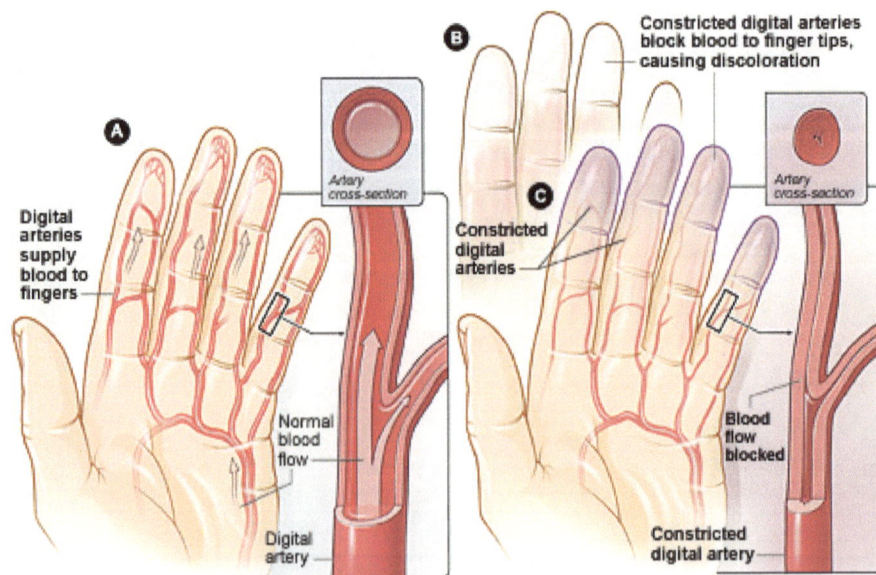

Figure 5.10 Raynaud's Phenomenon.

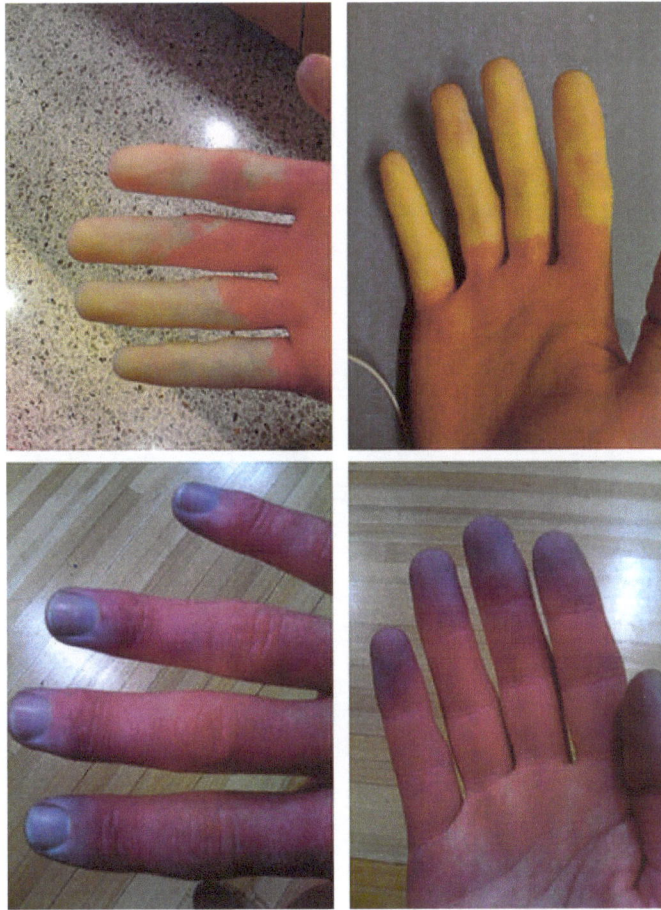

Figure 5.11 Discoloration of the Fingers.

I. Basic Physiology

● Smaller arteries that supply blood to the skin become narrow, limiting blood circulation. Over time, the arteries may begin to thicken, which limits the blood flow even further.

● Blood vessels normally constrict (narrow) in these areas in response to cold weather and emotional stress, but in cases of Raynaud's, this response is exaggerated.

● Common causes

  ○ Scleroderma

  ○ Systemic lupus erythematosus

  ○ Rheumatoid arthritis

  ○ Atherosclerosis

  ○ Arterial occlusive disease

  ○ Repetitive motion injury

  - ○ Drugs:
    - ▶ Amphetamines
    - ▶ Nicotine
    - ▶ Certain types of beta-blockers
    - ▶ Certain chemotherapy agents
    - ▶ Oral contraceptives

II. Clinical Signs and Symptoms

- Feeling of coldness or numbness in the extremities, often brought on by cold temperatures or emotional stress
- Discoloration of the fingers or toes
- Often the skin first turns white, then blue.
- As blood begins to flow normally again, the skin may turn red.
- May experience pain or tingling as circulation improves

III. Diagnostic Work-up

- Ultrasound used to identify blockages and examine blood vessel width

IV. Treatment

- Evaluate suspected underlying cause if any.
- Compare both sides of body, including blood pressure and pulse.
- Provide warmth and protection of affected extremities.
- Advise patient to avoid rapidly changing temperatures/environments.
- Risk for infection is high.
- Gloves should be worn when skin is at risk of trauma.
- If symptoms are severe, vasodilator drugs may be prescribed (to make the blood vessels relax)
  - ○ Nifedipine sustained release 30 mg/day; or
  - ○ Diltiazem sustained release 30 mg/day
- Aspirin is recommended if the patient is at risk of blood clot formation.
- If possible, the patient should stop taking any drugs listed under "Common causes," above.
- Stop smoking.

- Avoid caffeine.

V. Complications

- Skin ulcers: sores develop on the skin
- Infection
- Gangrene: tissue death due to lack of blood supply and oxygen

References

McPhee, Stephen J., and Papadakis, Maxine A. (2008). *Current Medical Diagnosis and Treatment 2010* (49th ed.). New York: McGraw-Hill Medical.

Raynaud's Disease. Mayo Clinic.
www.mayoclinic.org/diseases-conditions/raynauds-disease/multimedia/raynauds-disease/img-20005860

Figure 5.10 Raynaud's Phenomenon. Source: National Heart, Lung, and Blood Institute; National Institutes of Health; U.S. Department of Health and Human Services / What Is Raynaud's? Public Domain. Image at www.nhlbi.nih.gov/health/health-topics/topics/raynaud

Figure 5.11 Discoloration of the Fingers. Source: Tcal, File:Raynaud's syndrome.jpg, CC-BY-SA-3.0 / GNU Free Documentation. Image at commons.wikimedia.org/wiki/File:Raynaud%27s_Syndrome.jpg

Pericarditis

By Marian M. Houtman

Introduction

- Pericarditis refers to swelling and irritation of the pericardium, the membrane, or sac, that surrounds the heart.

- **Acute pericarditis** manifests as a sudden onset of chest pain.

  - Symptoms last no longer than a week.

- **Chronic pericarditis** manifests as subtle symptoms that begin gradually.

  - Usually lasts longer than six months

  - More common in men, 20 to 50 years of age

- Common causes of pericarditis include:

  - Idiopathic (unknown cause) in many cases

  - Viral infection (influenza A and B, measles, mumps)

  - Bacterial infection (tuberculosis or other bacteria)

  - Inflammatory disease (rheumatoid arthritis, scleroderma, sarcoidosis)

  - Other conditions: kidney failure, AIDS, cancer (lung or breast cancer most common)

  - Can develop after a heart attack (Dressler's syndrome) or invasive heart surgery

I. Anatomical Points

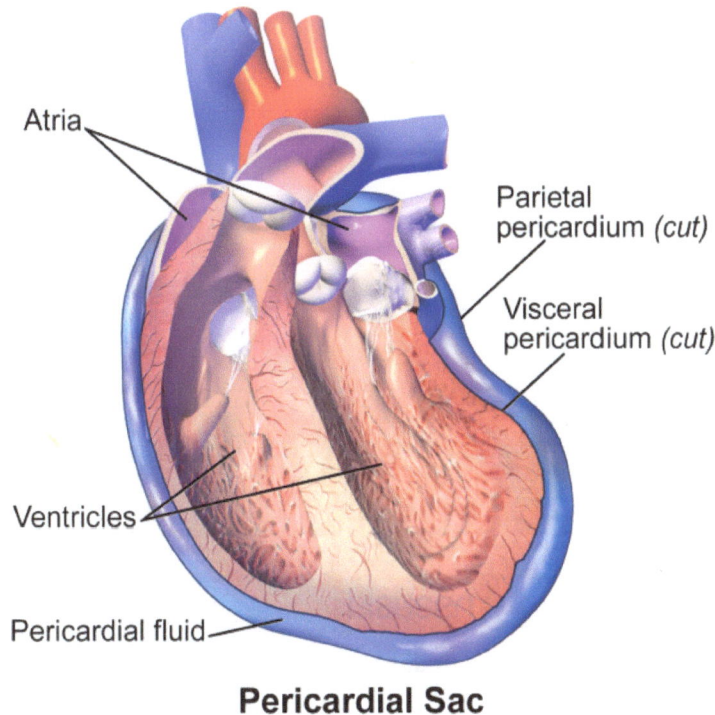

Atria

Parietal pericardium *(cut)*

Visceral pericardium *(cut)*

Ventricles

Pericardial fluid

Pericardial Sac

Figure 5.12 The Pericardial Sac, a Two-Layered Membrane Surrounding the Heart. The membranes contain a small amount of fluid between them allowing friction-free movement of the heart as it pumps.

II. Basic Physiology

- The pericardium is a sac-like membrane surrounding the heart (Figure 5.12).

- The pericardium is made up of two layers, with a gap between the layers that is filled with fluid.

- Pain associated with pericarditis is caused by irritated or inflamed layers of the sac rubbing against each other.

- The fluid between the layers can build up, resulting in an excessive amount, which puts pressure on the heart and decreases functioning.

III. Clinical Signs and Symptoms

- Sharp, piercing pain over left side of chest, neck or shoulder

- Shortness of breath when lying down

- Low-grade fever

- Feeling of weakness, fatigue, or anxiety
- Feeling sick
- Dry cough
- Abdominal or leg swelling

IV. Diagnostic Work-up

- Symptoms and recent medical history
- Perform physical assessment and take vital signs to look for these major indicators:
  - ○ Sharp pain in chest/back of shoulders
  - ○ Difficulty breathing
  - ○ Pain that often increases with deep breathing and lying flat, but lessens when the patient leans forward or sits in an upright position.
  - ○ Pain that increases with coughing and swallowing
  - ○ Listen with a stethoscope for "pericardial rub," a rubbing or creaking sound caused by the inflamed linings rubbing against each other.
- Ask about recent infection or heart attack, and obtain disease history.
- X-ray may show enlarged heart due to excess fluid accumulation in the pericardium.
- Electrocardiogram (EKG/ECG) can distinguish between pericarditis and myocardial infarction.
  - ○ ST segment changes are seen in all or most leads in pericarditis.
    - ▶ **Acute pericarditis**: usually concave ST segment (smiley face) *without* ST segment depression in leads opposite to those showing ST elevation (Figure 5.13)
    - ▶ **Acute MI**: usually convex, bowing upward *with* ST segment depression in leads opposite to those showing ST elevation (Figure 5.14)

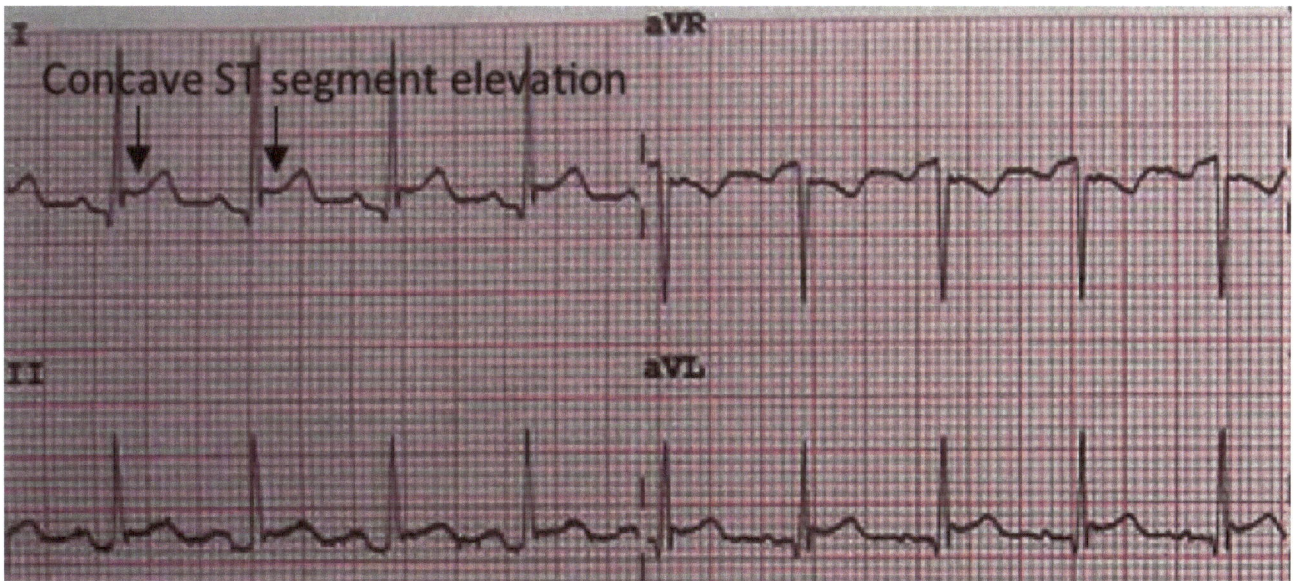

Figure 5.13 EKG Showing Pericarditis. Note the concave ST segment elevation. ST elevation will be present in most leads.

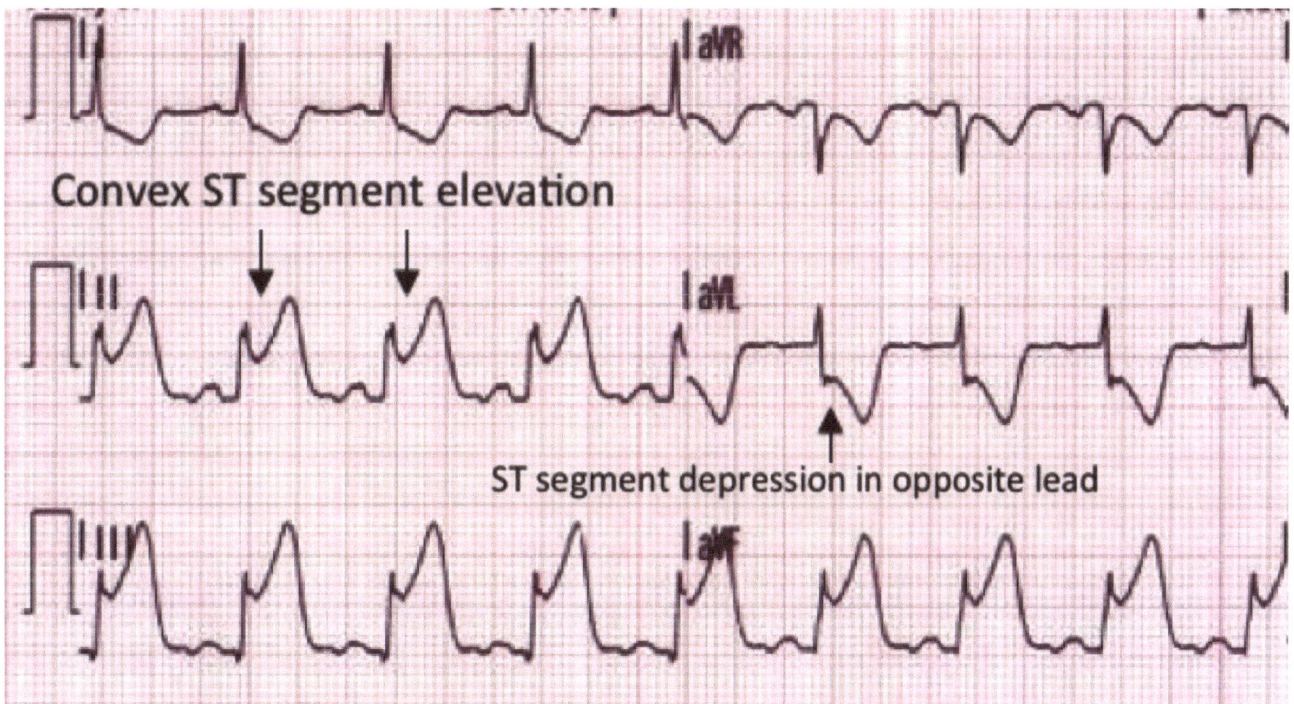

Figure 5.14 EKG Showing Acute MI. Note the convex ST segment elevation and the ST depression in the opposite lead.

V. Differential Diagnoses

- Pericarditis symptoms are similar to several heart and lung conditions.
- Pulmonary embolus (blood clot to the lung) and heart attack must be ruled out.

VI. Treatment

- Treatment depends on the cause, if known. Mild cases get better without treatment.
- Medications to reduce pain and inflammation:
  - Non-prescription: aspirin, ibuprofen
  - If pain is severe: short-term pain relief with a narcotic, such as morphine
  - Colchicines (Colcrys): this drug reduces inflammation, and can reduce duration of symptoms. This drug cannot be used if the patient has underlying health issues, such as liver or kidney disease.
  - Corticosteroids: may be used if the above medications are not effective.
    - If bacterial infection is determined to be the cause of the pericarditis, antibiotic therapy is required.
    - Drainage of the excess fluid may be necessary.

VII. Complications

- Uncontrolled chest pain
- Breathing difficulty
- Cardiac tamponade: excess fluid between the layers of the pericardium, preventing the proper functioning of the heart. *This is a medical emergency*.
  - Signs of cardiac tamponade (Beck's triad of symptoms):
    - Low blood pressure
    - Distended neck veins
    - Muffled heart sounds
  - Fluid can be drained using a sterile needle, with catheter attached, inserted through the chest wall into the pericardial sac (pericardiocentesis procedure).
  - The patient is monitored with EKG during the procedure.
- Constrictive pericarditis: long-term inflammation and recurrent pericarditis can cause permanent thickening, scarring, and contraction of the pericardium.
  - Pericardium becomes rigid, tightening around the heart, and preventing the heart from pumping properly.

- ○ Symptoms
  - ▶ Swelling of the legs and abdomen
  - ▶ Shortness of breath
- ○ May be treated medically initially, but may ultimately require surgery.
  - ▶ Pericardiectomy, which is full or partial removal of the pericardium.

References

Pericarditis. Cleveland Clinic. my.clevelandclinic.org/heart/disorders/other/pericarditis.aspx

Pericarditis. eMedicineHealth. emedicinehealth.com/pericarditis/page4_em.htm

Pericarditis. Mayo Clinic. www.mayoclinic.com/health/pericarditis/DS00505

Techniques: Heart Sounds and Murmurs. University of Washington. depts.washington.edu/physdx/heart/tech5.html

Figure 5.12 The Pericardial Sac, a Two-Layered Membrane Surrounding the Heart. Source: Blausen Medical Communications, Inc. Donated via OTRS / Wikimedia Commons / CC-BY-SA-3.0. Image at commons.wikimedia.org/wiki/File:Blausen_0724_PericardialSac.png

Figure 5.13 EKG Showing Pericarditis. Source: James Heilman, MD / Wikimedia Commons / CC-BY-SA-3.0 / GNU Free Documentation License. Image at en.wikipedia.org/wiki/File:Pericarditis10.JPG

Figure 5.14 EKG Showing Acute MI. Source: Glenlarson / Wikimedia Commons / Public Domain. Image at commons.wikimedia.org/wiki/File:12_lead_generated_inferior_MI.JPG

Tables

Table 1.1 Causes of Chest Pain 31

Table 1.2
Signs and Symptoms of Potentially Life-Threatening Causes of Chest Pain 36

Table 2.1 Differential Diagnoses for Acute Coronary Syndrome 52

Table 2.2 Medication for Suspected Angina 60

Table 2.3 Cardiac Lab Tests 63

Table 2.4 Cutoffs and Ranges for Troponin Types, 12 Hours After Onset of Pain 63

Table 2.5 Other Significant Blood Tests 64

Table 2.6 Laboratory Tests 71

Table 2.7 Drugs Used for MI: Dosing, Action, and Side Effects/Contraindications 74

Table 2.8 Blood Electrolyte Levels 92

Table 2.9 Tests for Kidney and Liver Function 93

Table 2.10 Treatment for Congestive Heart Failure 94

Table 3.1 Common Causes and Risk Factors for BBB 108

Table 3.2 Pharmaceutical Treatment Options for SVT 120

Table 3.3 Medication Options for Atrial Fibrillation 134

Table 3.4 Antiarrhythmic Drugs Used in the Treatment of Atrial Flutter 142

Table 3.5 Calcium Channel Blockers, Cardiac Glycosides, and Beta Blockers
Used in the Treatment of Atrial Flutter 144

Table 3.6
Anticoagulant and Antiplatelet Agents Used in the Treatment of Atrial Flutter 146

Table 3.7
Pharmaceutical Treatment Options for Wolff–Parkinson–White Syndrome 154

Table 3.8 Pharmaceutical Treatment Options for PVCs 161

Table 3.9 Pharmaceutical Treatment Options for Ventricular Tachycardia 169

Table 3.10 Pharmaceutical Treatment Options for Torsades de Pointes 181

Table 4.1 Characteristics of Varicose Veins 194

Table 5.1 Classification of Blood Pressure in Adults 209

Table 5.2 Typical Initial Prescription for Hypertensive Patients 210

Table 5.3 Recommended Medication for Adults (Age ≥18)
without Compelling Indications 211

Table 5.4 Antihypertensive Agents and Adverse Effects 213

Table 5.5 Dosing Guidelines for Vancomycin in Infective Endocarditis
with Unconfirmed Pathogen 221

Table 5.6 Treatment for Infectious Endocarditis Caused by Streptococci 222

Table 5.7 Treatment for Infectious Endocarditis Caused by Enterococci 222

Table 5.8 Treatment for Infectious Endocarditis Caused by Staphylococci 222

Table 5.9 Treatment for Infectious Endocarditis Caused by HACEK* Organisms 223

Table 5.10 Interpretation of Ankle Brachial Pressure Index (ABPI) 233

Table 5.11 Pharmaceutical Treatment Options for PAD 234

About the Editors

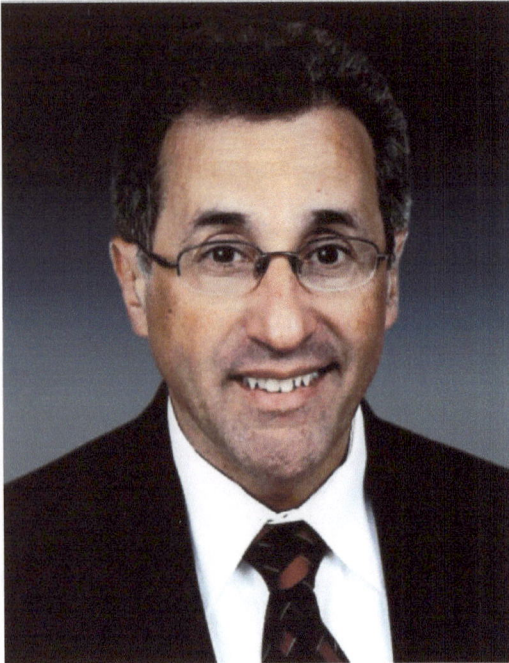

Dr. Robert Simon founded International Medical Corps in 1984 in response to the need for medical services and training inside war-torn Afghanistan. A renowned expert in Emergency Medicine, Dr. Simon is the author of numerous textbooks on orthopedic emergencies and surgical procedures, which are used as standards in Emergency Medicine throughout the United States. Dr. Simon is a professor in the Department of Emergency Medicine at Rush University, Stroger-Cook County Hospital in Chicago, Illinois. He is also former Bureau Chief of the Cook County Bureau of Health Services. He serves as Chairman of the Board of International Medical Corps.

Dr. Henry Hood is among the earliest International Medical Corps volunteers. An orthopedic surgeon in Lancaster, Ohio, Dr. Hood joined in 1985 to fulfill the organization's mission in the war in Afghanistan and in the refugee camps of Pakistan. In response to the need in Afghanistan, Dr. Hood solved a major medical problem of resource-poor environments, designing a traction system made out of wooden poles and rope that could be duplicated anywhere in the world. He has also volunteered in Somalia, Indonesia, and Haiti, among others. Dr. Hood has served as the Associate Board Chair of International Medical Corps since 1988.

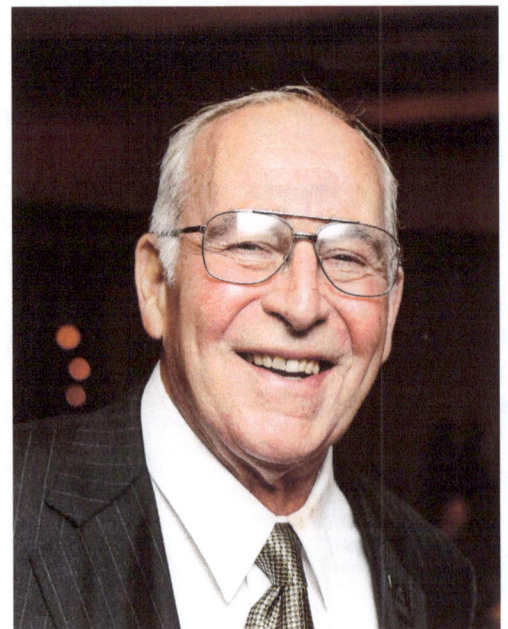

Master Table
of Contents

Preface   16

Unit 1: Cardiology   19

  1 Introduction to Cardiology

  2 Cardiac Diseases and Disorders

  3 Arrhythmias

  4 Venous Disease

  5 Other Cardiovascular Conditions

Unit 2: Dermatology, Immunology, and Allergic Disorders   249

  6 Introduction to Dermatological Disorders

  7 Common Dermatological Conditions

  8 Bacterial Skin Infections

  9 Fungal Skin Infections

  10 Parasitic Skin Infections

  11 Viral Skin Diseases

  12 Nail Disorders

13 Benign Tumors

14 Immunology and Allergic Disorders

Unit 3: Endocrine and Metabolic Disorders   407

15 Overview of Endocrine and Metabolic Disorders

16 Thyroid Diseases

17 Adrenal Gland Dysfunction

18 Blood Sugar Disorders

Unit 4: Ear, Nose, Throat, and Dental Disorders   457

19 Introduction to ENT Disorders

20 Approach to the Patient with Ear Problems

21 Diseases and Disorders of the Nose and Throat

22 ENT Foreign Bodies

23 Dental Diseases and Disorders

Unit 5: Genitourinary and Renal Disorders   643

24 Common Genitourinary Complaints

25 Renal and Urinary System Disorders

26 Disorders Specific to the Male Genitourinary System

Unit 6: Gastrointestinal Disorders   769

27 Overview of Painful GI Complaints

28 Gastrointestinal Diseases and Disorders

29 Anorectal Disorders

30 Hepatic and Biliary Disorders

Unit 7: Hematology and Oncology 985

31 Introduction to Hematology

32 Overview of Anemia Types

33 Hematology and Oncology Diseases and Disorders

Unit 8: Infectious Disease 1069

34 Overview of Infectious Disease

35 Infectious Diseases

Unit 9: Neurology 1319

36 Anatomy and Physiology of the Brain and CNS

37 Approach to the Neurological Patient

38 Overview of Common Neurological Symptoms

39 Neurological Diseases and Disorders

Unit 10: Nursing Care 1463

40 Core Principles of Nursing

41 Basic Nursing Care

42 Advanced Nursing Care

Unit 11: Gynecology and Obstetrics 1579

43 Gynocological Assessment

44 Breast Diseases and Conditions

45 OB/GYN Disorders and Procedures

Unit 12: Ophthalmology   1757

46 Introduction to the Eye

47 Review of Common Ophthalmic Complaints

48 Disorders of the Eye

49 Orbital Diseases

50 Traumatic Ophthalmic Injuries

51 Penetrating and Perforating Injury to the Eyeball

52 Trauma of the Eyelids, Orbit, and Adjacent Structures

Unit 13: Orthopedics   1909

53 Comprehensive Approach to the Orthopedic Patient

54 Joint Disorders

55 Crystal-Induced Arthritis

56 Infections of Joints and Bones

57 Bursitis, Tendinitis, and Fibromyalgia

58 Hand Disorders

59 Wrist Disorders

60 Elbow Disorders

61 Shoulder and Arm Disorders

62 Hip Disorders

63 Knee Disorders

64 Leg Disorders

65 Foot and Ankle Disorders

Unit 14: Pediatrics   2313

66 General Care of Infants and Children

67 Pediatric Diseases and Disorders

Unit 15: Pharmacology   2477

68 Introduction to Pharmacology

69 Drug Categories

Unit 16: Pulmonary Disorders   2711

70 Pulmonary Diseases and Disorders

71 Mediastinal and Pleural Disorders

Unit 17: Tropical Medicine   2797

72 Tropical Diseases and Disorders

Guide to Tables   2975

About the Editors   2999

www.ingramcontent.com/pod-product-compliance
Lightning Source LLC
Chambersburg PA
CBHW050823220326
41598CB00006B/305